ENDOMORPH

TRANSFORMATION

The Ultimate Guide to
Building Lean Muscle and Boosting Metabolism.

LOLAH JOHNSON

Copyright © 2023 by **Lolah Johnson**

All rights reserved.

No part of this book may be used or reproduced in any form whatsoever without written permission except in the case of brief quotations in critical articles or reviews.

Printed in the United States of America.

First Edition: MAY 2023

TABLE OF CONTENT

INTRODUCTION

First, I'd like to thank you for selecting this book. I hope you found it useful and informative.

Understanding the Endomorph Body Type Definition and Characteristics of Endomorphs

Endomorphs, along with ectomorphs and mesomorphs, are one of the three basic body forms identified by William Sheldon in the 1940s. Endomorphs tend to have a larger amount of body fat and a rounder, softer look than the other body types.

The following characteristics typically serve to identify endomorphs:

Body Composition: Endomorphs have a predisposition to accumulate fat quickly, particularly in the lower belly, hips, and thighs.

They often have greater bone structure and a softer, curvier body.

Slower Metabolism: Endomorphs have a slower metabolic rate, which means their bodies may burn calories at a slower rate. This might make losing weight or maintaining a lean body composition more difficult.

Difficulty Losing Weight: Endomorphs may find it more difficult to shed weight than other body types due to their genetic tendency. To reach their ideal physique, they may need to put in more work and use certain tactics.

Higher Fat Storage: Endomorphs have a stronger tendency to retain extra calories as body fat, which can make it harder to achieve a slim and defined appearance. It is critical that they focus on maintaining a healthy balance of calorie intake and expenditure.

Muscular Potential: Endomorphs may have a tougher difficulty reducing fat, but they often have the capacity to produce powerful and well-developed muscles. They may obtain a lean and toned figure with the appropriate exercise and nutrition.

It's crucial to remember that body types exist on a continuum, and people might have traits from different body types to varied degrees. Understanding one's body type can aid in adjusting training and diet strategies to attain the best outcomes.

Body Composition and Metabolism Considerations

Endomorphs' particular traits necessitate careful evaluation of body composition and metabolism. Here are some key items to remember:

Body Fat Percentage: Endomorphs often have a greater body fat percentage when compared to other body types. This implies individuals have more adipose tissue, which might have an impact on their total body composition and aesthetic aspirations.

Muscle Mass: Endomorphs have the ability to gain substantial muscular mass. Despite their naturally stockier shape, their bodies adapt well to strength and resistance training. By boosting calorie expenditure, lean muscle can assist raise metabolism and improve body composition.

Basal Metabolic Rate (BMR): Endomorphs frequently have a somewhat lower basal metabolic rate, which is the quantity of calories the body requires to execute fundamental tasks at rest. This implies they may require less calories than others with greater metabolic rates. Caloric intake can be adjusted to aid with weight control and fat loss objectives.

Metabolic Adaptation: Endomorphs may experience metabolic adaptation, in which the body adjusts to a decreasing calorie intake over time. Weight reduction may become more difficult as the body grows more effective at preserving energy. Adjusting calorie intake on a regular basis or integrating strategic refeed days might help prevent this adaptation.

Nutrient Sensitivity: Endomorphs may be more sensitive to specific nutrients, such as carbs, than other types of people. Some endomorphs find that cutting carbs and focusing on greater protein and moderate fat consumption might help them lose fat. Individual differences and tastes, however, should be taken into account when calculating the optimal macronutrient ratios.

It is critical to handle body composition and metabolic issues in a tailored manner. A registered dietitian or certified fitness expert who specializes in working with endomorphs can give specific advice and methods to enhance body composition and promote metabolic health.

Challenges faced by Endomorphs in building Lean Muscle and Boosting Metabolism.

Increased propensity to accumulate body fat

Endomorphs are more likely than other body types to retain body fat. This is due to a combination of variables such as heredity, hormonal impacts, and metabolic variances. Here are some major concerns about endomorphs' increased proclivity to accumulate body fat:

Fat Storage Areas: Endomorphs frequently store fat in certain parts of the body, such as the lower belly, hips, and thighs. These areas contain a larger concentration of fat cells and are more likely to store fat. Endomorphs must concentrate on specific workouts and a complete training regimen that covers these areas.

Hormonal Factors: Hormones have an important role in fat accumulation and metabolic regulation.

Endomorphs' hormone patterns may encourage fat accumulation. They may, for example, have greater estrogen levels, which can lead to increased fat deposition, particularly in the lower body.

Metabolic Rate: Endomorphs frequently have a slower metabolic rate, which means their bodies burn calories at a slower rate. This can make creating a calorie deficit for weight reduction more difficult. They may need to be more conscious of their calorie intake and consume an adequate amount to support their goals.

Insulin Sensitivity: Endomorphs may have lower insulin sensitivity, which affects how effectively their bodies consume and retain carbs. This can result in greater variations in blood sugar levels and perhaps increased fat accumulation. Managing carbohydrate consumption, emphasizing complex carbohydrates, and avoiding excess sugar can all assist to regulate insulin levels.

Balanced Nutrition: Endomorphs must have a well-balanced and healthy diet. Prioritizing complete, unprocessed meals, lean proteins, fiber-rich carbs, and healthy fats can help with satiety, calorie control, and general health. Balancing macronutrients and adopting portion control can also aid in the management of body fat.

While endomorphs are more likely to accumulate body fat, it's important to remember that a variety of factors, including genetics, nutrition, activity, and lifestyle, affect body composition. Endomorphs can attain their chosen body composition objectives and enhance their general health and well-being with a personalized approach to nutrition and exercise.

Having trouble reducing weight and developing muscle

Because of their particular body composition and metabolic features, endomorphs frequently have difficulties in both reducing weight and developing muscle. Here are some things to think about:

1. Challenges for Weight Loss:

- **Slower Metabolism:** Endomorphs often have a slower metabolic rate, which can make creating the calorie deficit required for weight reduction more difficult. They may need to be more conscious of their calorie intake and alter it more than people with quicker metabolisms.

- **Fat Storage:** Endomorphs have a higher proclivity to retain fat, particularly in troublesome places such as the belly, hips, and thighs. This can make it more difficult to lose body fat in particular regions, necessitating a tailored strategy with a combination of good nutrition and activity.

- **Insulin Sensitivity:** Endomorphs may have lower insulin sensitivity, which makes it simpler to retain extra carbs as fat. It is critical to focus on a well-balanced diet that prioritizes complex carbs, lean proteins, and healthy fats.

2. Considerations for Muscle Gain:

- **Potential for Muscle Growth:** Endomorphs frequently have a genetic edge when it comes to growing muscle. They have a larger frame and may grow powerful, well-defined muscles. Resistance training with increasing loading is vital for encouraging muscle growth and reaching the body of your dreams.

- **Muscle Building Nutrition:** Endomorphs should consume enough protein to assist muscle repair and development. Adequate calorie intake, including a macronutrient balance, is essential for providing the energy needed for exercises and promoting muscle growth.

- **Balanced Training Program:** A well-designed strength training program that incorporates compound exercises, isolation exercises, and enough rest and recovery times is essential for maximum muscular growth. Consistency and gradual loading are essential for keeping the muscles challenged and growing.

Endomorphs must take a comprehensive strategy that includes tailored nutrition, good workout regimens, and a constant and patient mentality.

Working with a trained fitness expert or nutritionist who knows endomorphs' unique needs can give individualized direction and assistance in reaching weight reduction and muscle growth objectives.

Slower metabolic rate and potential hormonal factors

Endomorphs frequently have a slower metabolic rate than other body types, which can make weight reduction and muscle building more difficult. Here's a closer look at endomorphs' slower metabolic rate and possibly hormonal factors:

1. Metabolic Rate Slower:

- **Basal Metabolic Rate (BMR):** Endomorphs often have a lower BMR, which is the quantity of calories the body requires at rest to execute fundamental processes. This means individuals naturally burn less calories throughout the day, making creating a calorie deficit for weight reduction more challenging.

- **Energy Expenditure**: Endomorphs should be aware of their entire energy expenditure, which includes physical activity levels and exercise. Regular physical exercise, such as cardio and weight training, can assist to increase total calorie burn and metabolic rate over time.

2. Hormonal Aspects:

- **Estrogen:** Endomorphs may have greater estrogen levels, a hormone that influences fat accumulation and distribution. Elevated estrogen levels can lead to increased fat accumulation in certain places such as the hips and thighs.
- **Insulin Sensitivity:** Endomorphs may also have decreased insulin sensitivity, which affects how well the body processes and

uses carbs. Poor insulin sensitivity can result in elevated circulating insulin levels and an increased probability of fat accumulation.

Cortisol: Stress has been shown to impact hormone levels, notably cortisol, often known as the stress hormone. Cortisol levels that are chronically raised can contribute to increased fat accumulation, particularly in the abdomen area.

The following measures can be used to manage hormonal variables and promote a healthy metabolic rate:

Balanced Nutrition: Eating a well-balanced diet rich in nutrient-dense foods will assist maintain normal hormone levels and metabolism. Consume lots of whole grains, lean proteins, healthy fats, and fruits and vegetables.

Strength Training: Including strength training activities on a regular basis can assist increase muscle mass and metabolic rate. Resistance workouts help to build muscle and burn calories both during and after a workout.

Stress Reduction: Stress-relieving practices such as mindfulness, meditation, and regular exercise can help control cortisol levels and reduce its influence on metabolism and fat accumulation.

While endomorphs have additional obstacles due to slower metabolic rates and hormonal considerations, a well-rounded strategy that includes correct diet, frequent exercise, and stress management can assist improve weight loss and muscle growth efforts. It is critical to get specific counsel geared to individual needs from healthcare specialists or qualified fitness gurus.

Strength training is essential for Endomorphs.

Role of strength training in body composition transformation

Strength training is essential for body composition change, especially for endomorphs aiming to gain lean muscle and enhance their overall physique. Here are some of the reasons why strength training is so important:

Muscle Development: Strength training is intended to target and activate muscular fibers, resulting in muscle hypertrophy (growth) over time. Endomorphs can enhance their muscle mass by indulging in regular strength training activities, which not only improves their strength and performance but also adds to a more defined and sculpted body.

Increased Metabolic Rate: Strength training helps build lean muscle, which boosts metabolism. Muscles are metabolically active tissues, which means that they burn more calories at rest than fat tissue. Endomorphs can increase their basal metabolic rate (BMR) and calorie expenditure even when they are not actively exercising by increasing muscle mass. This can help with weight loss and enhance body composition.

Fat reduction: Strength training has been shown to directly contribute to fat reduction. Endomorphs produce a stimulation that stimulates energy expenditure when they engage in resistance activities. When paired with a proper diet, this results in a calorie deficit, which is necessary for decreasing body fat. Strength training also helps to maintain lean muscle mass during weight reduction, ensuring that the bulk of weight lost is from fat rather than muscle tissue.

Body Shape and Definition: By targeting particular muscle areas, strength training helps shape and define the body. Endomorphs can increase muscle and improve overall body form by focusing on activities that target their problem regions, such as the lower belly, hips, and thighs. Squats and deadlifts, for example, utilize several muscle groups and produce a balanced physique.

Strength and Functional Fitness: Strength training improves not only appearance but also functional fitness. Endomorphs can execute daily activities more effectively, lower the chance of injury, and improve overall physical performance by boosting muscle strength.

Endomorphs should consider the following to optimize the effects of strength training for body composition transformation:

Consistency: Regularity and consistency in strength training sessions are essential for getting desired outcomes. Aim for at least two to three sessions of strength training every week. **Progressive Overload:** Gradually increase the intensity, volume, or complexity of workouts over time to keep the muscles challenged and growing.

perfect Form and Technique: To reduce the chance of injury and maximize muscle activation, focus on completing exercises with perfect form and technique.

Balanced Training Program: To promote total muscular growth and balance, include a combination of complex exercises (targeting many muscle groups) and isolation exercises (targeting individual muscles).

Allow enough rest and recovery time between strength training sessions to allow the muscles to rebuild and expand.

Strength training, along with correct diet and aerobic activity, can have a transformational effect on body composition for endomorphs, resulting in greater muscle tone, higher metabolism, and a more attractive body shape.

Muscle building and Metabolism Enhancement benefits

Strength training has several advantages for muscle gain and metabolic enhancement. Here are the main benefits:

Muscular Hypertrophy: Strength training stimulates muscular development. Resistance workouts, such as weightlifting and bodyweight exercises, cause tiny damage to your muscle fibers. As a result of this injury, your body begins the process of muscle repair and growth, which results in muscular hypertrophy. Consistent strength training can lead to increased muscle growth and definition over time.

Increased Metabolic Rate: Strength training helps you build lean muscle mass, which boosts your metabolism. Muscles are metabolically active tissues, which means they require energy (calories) even while resting. Your basal metabolic rate (BMR) increases when you grow muscle, resulting in a greater calorie expenditure throughout the day. This can help with weight loss and make it simpler to maintain a healthy body weight.

Calorie Expenditure: Strength exercise burns calories on its own. While it may not burn as many calories as aerobic activities, strength training stimulates your muscles and demands energy to complete. This might lead to an increase in calorie expenditure during and after your exercises as your body strives to heal and rebuild the muscles.

Fat reduction and Body Composition: Strength training is important for fat reduction and body composition improvement. Your body gets more effective at burning fat as you gain lean muscle mass. Muscle tissue is more metabolically active than fat tissue and takes more energy to maintain. As a result, the more muscle you have, the more calories your body burns at rest, potentially contributing to weight loss.

Hormonal Benefits: Strength exercise can have a good impact on hormone levels, notably testosterone and growth hormone, which are important for muscle development and repair. These hormones not only aid with muscle growth, but also with metabolism and fat burning.

Functional Strength and Performance: Strength training promotes not just muscle size but also strength, power, and functional fitness. This can help you do daily activities, sports, and physical duties more easily and efficiently. It can also aid in the prevention of age-related muscle loss and the maintenance of independence as you age.

Consider the following suggestions to optimize the muscle-building and metabolism-boosting effects of strength training:

Progressive Overload: Keep your muscles challenged by gradually increasing the resistance, intensity, or volume of your workouts. This promotes more muscle development and adaptability.

Balanced Training Program: Incorporate a range of workouts that target different muscle groups to guarantee total muscular growth and balance.

Sufficient Protein Consumption: Consume enough high-quality protein to assist muscle repair and development. Aim for 0.7 to 1 gram of protein per pound of body weight every day.

Rest and recovery: Give your muscles enough time between strength training sessions to recuperate and repair. Getting proper sleep and implementing rest days into your fitness plan are two examples.

Maintain and build on your success by engaging in strength training activities on a consistent basis, aiming for at least two to three sessions each   week.

higher muscle mass, improved metabolism, higher fat reduction, and functional strength can all be obtained by combining strength training into your exercise regimen. Remember to work with a fitness professional or trainer to create a program that is tailored to your specific objectives and fitness level.

Positive impact on overall health and well-being

Strength training has a significant influence on general health and well-being in addition to the specialized advantages for muscle growth and metabolic enhancement. Here are some of the ways strength training may benefit your overall health:

Bone Health: Strength training is a weight-bearing exercise that promotes bone density and strength. It has been shown to lower the risk of osteoporosis and age-related bone loss in postmenopausal women and older individuals.

Joint Health and Injury Prevention: Strength exercise, by strengthening the muscles around your joints, can give improved support and stability, lowering the chance of injuries and joint-related issues. It also helps with joint flexibility and range of motion.

Posture and Alignment: Strength training exercises target particular muscle groups, including those involved in posture and alignment. Strength training can assist improve posture and minimize muscular imbalances by strengthening the muscles in your back, core, and shoulders.

Mental Health and Cognitive Function: Regular strength training improves mental health and cognitive function. It can help reduce anxiety and depression symptoms, increase mood, promote self-esteem, and improve general psychological well-being. Strength training has also been linked to better cognitive function, such as memory and concentration.

Chronic Disease Management: Strength training can help in the management and prevention of chronic illnesses. It has been demonstrated that it improves insulin sensitivity, glucose metabolism, and blood lipid profiles. It can also aid in the reduction of blood pressure and the risk of cardiovascular disease.

Functional Independence: Strength training enhances functional fitness, which refers to the capacity to do daily chores with ease and independence. Strength training can improve your capacity to carry out everyday tasks, retain mobility, and lower your risk of falling by developing muscle strength, endurance, and flexibility.

Longevity and Aging: Strength training has been linked to greater lifespan and a higher quality of life as you become older. It contributes to the preservation of muscle mass, bone density, and functional capacities, lowering the risk of age-related deterioration and frailty.

Stress Reduction: Strength training, like any other kind of exercise, may be an excellent stress reliever. It stimulates the production of endorphins, which are natural mood-enhancing substances in the brain that aid in stress relief, relaxation, and general mental well-being.

Strength training must be done consistently and in conjunction with other healthy lifestyle choices such as right diet, aerobic activity, and enough rest and recovery to have a beneficial influence on overall health and well-being. Remember to begin slowly, listen to your body, and get the advice of a healthcare practitioner or fitness expert if you have any special health issues or illnesses.

CHAPTER ONE
FUNDAMENTALS OF STRENGTH TRAINING FOR ENDOMORPHS

Fundamentals of successful Strength Training

Progressive overload for muscle stimulation

Progressive overload is a key strength-training strategy that entails gradually increasing the demands imposed on your muscles over time. You encourage greater muscle growth and strength development by continually testing your muscles with progressively higher levels of resistance. Here is how progressive overload works and how to use it effectively:

Increasing Resistance: Increasing the resistance or weight raised throughout your workouts is the most popular approach to applying progressive overload. As your muscles adapt to a certain weight, you must raise the resistance to keep them challenged. This may be accomplished by adding extra weight to the barbell, dumbbells, or workout machines you utilize. Bodyweight exercises may be made more challenging by utilizing resistance bands, adding weight vests, or moving to more complex forms.

Changing Repetitions and Sets: You may also use progressive overload by changing the number of repetitions and sets you do. You may increase the number of repetitions you execute with a particular weight as your muscles strengthen. For example, if you were performing 8 reps with a given weight at first, you may gradually raise it to 10 or 12 reps, and you can even add an extra set to your training regimen to enhance the overall volume and intensity.

Manipulation of Tempo and Time Under Tension: Tempo refers to the rate at which each repeat of an activity is performed. You can create varied challenges for your muscles by varying the tempo. Slowing down the eccentric (lowering) component of the exercise, for example, might increase the duration under strain and give a stronger stimulus for muscle development. Experiment with varied tempos and strategies to alter the input and keep moving forward.

Increasing Frequency and Training Volume: You may produce progressive overload by increasing the frequency and overall training volume. You can raise the frequency of training a muscle group to twice or three times per week instead of once per week. You may also raise the overall volume by executing additional exercises or sets for a single muscle group during a training session. To avoid overtraining, however, it is critical to balance frequency and volume with proper rest and recuperation.

Improving Technique and Range of Motion: Improving your workout technique and range of motion is another part of progressive overload. As you gain proficiency in a specific exercise, you may concentrate on improving your form and expanding your range of motion. This ensures that you are targeting the correct muscles and getting the most out of each workout.

Remember that increasing loading should be done gradually and carefully to enable your muscles, joints, and connective tissues to adapt and avoid injuries. Listen to your body, go at a rate that feels difficult but achievable, and always emphasize perfect form and technique.

You may assure continued muscle activation, development, and strength increases in your strength training regimen by constantly implementing the principle of progressive overload. Keep track of your progress, make modifications as needed, and celebrate your fitness achievements.

Proper rest and recovery for muscle repair and growth

A good strength training program requires enough rest and recuperation. They let your muscles recover and renew, which optimizes muscular growth and reduces the danger of overtraining. Here are some crucial considerations for optimal rest and recovery:

Adequate Sleep: A good night's sleep is essential for muscle repair and development. Your body produces growth hormone as you sleep, which aids in muscle healing. To ensure optimal recuperation, aim for 7-9 hours of uninterrupted sleep every night.

Rest Days: Include regular rest days in your training plan. Allow your muscles, joints, and neurological system to recover from the stress of hard exercises these days. Listen to your body and give yourself at least one or two days of total rest every week.

Active Recovery: Consider engaging in active recovery activities such as mild stretching, yoga, or low-intensity exercise on rest days. These activities increase blood flow, aid in the removal of metabolic waste products, and can aid in muscle repair.

Proper Nutrition: Proper nutrition is essential for muscle repair and development. Make sure you eat a well-balanced diet with enough protein, carbs, and healthy fats. Protein is extremely important since it serves as the foundation for muscle repair. Stay hydrated as well, and consider including post-workout meals or snacks that contain both protein and carbs to aid recuperation.

Stretching and Foam rolling: Stretching and foam rolling can help relieve muscular pain and increase flexibility. Foam rolling, in particular, may be used to target tight regions, relieve stress, and improve blood circulation. Include these techniques in your cool-down regimen after workouts or on days off.

Active Warm-ups: Perform a dynamic warm-up routine before beginning your exercises to prepare your muscles and joints for the next activity. Light aerobic workouts, mobility drills, and dynamic stretches can all be included. A proper warm-up improves blood flow and lowers the chance of injury.

Pay Attention to Your Body: Pay attention to your body's signals and modify your workout accordingly. If you have chronic muscular pain, exhaustion, or a drop in performance, it might be an indication that you need to rest more or do a lighter workout. Pushing through extreme exhaustion or discomfort might result in overtraining and injury.

Stress Management: Excessive stress can have a detrimental influence on your healing and muscle-building efforts. Include stress-reduction practices like meditation, deep breathing exercises, or hobbies that help you relax and unwind.

Remember that rest and recuperation are just as vital as exercise. Because everyone's recovery needs differ, it's critical to listen to your body and establish the proper mix of training intensity and recuperation time. By putting appropriate rest and recovery first, you allow your muscles to mend and get stronger, resulting in faster overall improvement on your strength training journey.

Workout adaptation and diversity for sustained improvement

Workout adaptation and diversity are critical for maintaining success on your strength training journey. When your body becomes acclimated to a specific training regimen, it adapts and becomes more efficient, slowing your development. Here are a few ideas for incorporating adaptability and variation into your workouts:

Progressive Overload: As previously said, progressive overload is required for continued advancement. To test your muscles and drive additional growth, gradually increase the intensity, volume, or complexity of your exercises. Over time, increase the weight you lift, the number of repetitions you do, or the number of sets you do.

Exercise Selection: Vary your workouts to target different muscle groups and activate them from various angles. In order to engage diverse muscles and promote general balance and growth, incorporate a combination of complex exercises (such as squats, deadlifts, and bench presses) and isolation exercises (such as bicep curls or calf raises).

Training Methods: Use a range of training methods to give diversity and challenge to your exercises. Supersets (doing two exercises back-to-back with a short recovery), drop sets (dropping weight after achieving muscular exhaustion to complete the set), and pyramids (gradually increasing or decreasing weight with each set) are examples of these. These approaches might help you break through plateaus and keep your training interesting.

Alter rep ranges and rest intervals: Vary your rep ranges and rest intervals in your exercises. For example, in one phase, you can focus on heavy weights and low repetitions for strength and power development and then move to moderate weights and higher repetitions for muscular endurance and hypertrophy in the next. Manipulate rest intervals in the same way to test your muscles differently and foster diverse energy systems.

Circuit Training and High-Intensity Interval Training (HIIT): Incorporate circuit training or high-intensity interval training (HIIT) into your program. These training methods involve alternating between various exercises or short bursts of intense activity and rest periods. They can increase cardiovascular fitness, burn calories, and give your muscles a fresh stimulus.

Periodization: Periodization is the process of methodically varying training variables such as volume, intensity, and frequency throughout set time intervals. This method aids in the prevention of plateaus, enhances rehabilitation, and maximizes long-term success. It usually entails segmenting your training into several phases, such as hypertrophy, strength, and peaking.

Cross-Training: Include different types of exercise and physical activities in your program. Yoga, Pilates, swimming, cycling, or athletics are examples of such activities. Cross-training allows you to work other muscle groups, improve your overall fitness, and take a mental break from your typical strength training program.

Mind-Muscle Connection: During exercises, concentrate on increasing your mind-muscle connection. Concentrate on the muscle regions you want to work on and do exercises with slow, controlled motions. This promotes improved overall muscular growth by ensuring good technique and maximizing muscle activation.

By introducing adaptability and variation into your exercises, you can keep your muscles challenged, avoid plateaus, and continue to improve your strength, muscular growth, and general fitness. Be willing to attempt new exercises, methods, and training styles, as well as listen to your body and modify the intensity and volume as needed. Consistency and constant growth are essential for establishing and maintaining long-term success.

Setting realistic goals and tracking progress

Defining specific, measurable goals for muscle gain and fat loss

Setting clear, quantifiable objectives is critical for tracking your progress and remaining motivated throughout your muscle growth and fat reduction journey. Here are some principles for developing clear, quantifiable, and successful goals:

Specific: Clearly explain your objectives. Instead of broad objectives like "gain muscle" or "lose fat," be precise about how much muscle you want to acquire or how much body fat you want to shed. For instance, you may aim to add 5 pounds of lean muscle or lower your body fat percentage by 3%.

quantifiable: Make sure your objectives are quantifiable so you can measure your progress and know when you've met them. Use measurable indicators such as body weight, body fat percentage, waist circumference, and muscle measurements. This allows you to objectively measure your progress and alter your strategy as needed.

Time-bound: Establish a timetable for achieving your objectives. A deadline fosters a sense of urgency and prevents procrastination. It also makes it easier to keep track of your development. For example, you may set a goal of gaining 5 pounds of lean muscle in three months or decreasing your body fat percentage by 3% in six weeks.

Realistic: Realistic objectives are those that are difficult but attainable. When assessing what is reasonable for you, consider your current fitness level, lifestyle, and responsibilities. Choosing too ambitious and difficult-to-attain objectives can be demotivating, while choosing goals that are too simple may not give enough of a challenge. Find the ideal balance that takes you out of your comfort zone while still being doable.

Break it Down: Divide your key goals into smaller, more doable milestones. This allows you to enjoy small victories along the way, which keeps you motivated and focused. For example, if your objective is to build 10 pounds of muscle in six months, you can aim for a monthly growth rate of 2 pounds of muscle.

Track Progress: Assess and track your progress toward your goals on a regular basis. To track progress, use tools such as body measurements, progress images, and performance indicators. This not only keeps you accountable, but it also allows you to make changes to your training and eating plan as needed.

Adjust and adapt: Be willing to change your goals as you get more information about your body's response. Your initial goals may need to be adjusted depending on your own circumstances and how your body responds to your workout and eating plan.

Remember that your objectives should be tailored to your own requirements, interests, and starting position. It's also crucial to focus on non-scale successes and other signs of improvement, such as greater strength, energy, or overall well-being.

Setting defined, quantifiable objectives for muscle building and fat loss gives you a clear path for your journey. It assists you in remaining motivated, tracking your progress, and making educated decisions along the way. Accept the process, be patient, and enjoy each step forward toward your goals.

Monitoring progress with metrics and measures

Metrics and measures are useful tools for tracking your progress while you build muscle and lose fat. They give objective statistics that can assist you in tracking your progress and making the required changes to your exercise and eating regimen. You can utilize the following essential metrics and measurements:

Body Weight: Weighing yourself on a reputable scale on a regular basis might provide you with an indication of your overall development. However, keep in mind that swings in body weight can be impacted by things like water retention and muscle building, so other metrics must be considered as well.

Body Composition: Measuring your body composition gives you a more precise view of your muscle mass and body fat percentage changes. Dual-energy X-ray absorptiometry

(DEXA) scans, bioelectrical impedance analysis (BIA), and skinfold caliper measures can all aid in determining the proportion of body fat and muscle mass.

Circumference Measurements: Measurements of certain body circumferences, such as the waist, hips, thighs, and arms, can aid in monitoring changes in body fat distribution. It's particularly effective for monitoring development in certain areas and assessing changes in body shape and composition.

Progress Photos: Before-and-after images taken at regular intervals allow you to clearly compare your physique over time. It assists you in detecting changes that may not be represented in statistics alone, such as improved muscle definition and overall body composition.

Metrics for Strength and Performance: Tracking your strength increases and performance enhancements may be a fantastic sign of success. Keep track of how much weight you lift, how many repetitions you do, and how long it takes you to finish various exercises. Increasing these measurements gradually reveals gains in muscular strength and endurance.

Energy Levels and Recovery: Assessing your energy levels and recuperation can provide you with insight into how well your body is adjusting to your training and diet strategy. Check to see whether you're feeling more energy, recovering faster between exercises, and overall feeling better.

Subjective Feelings and Body Awareness: Notice how you feel and how your body reacts to your workout and nourishment. Observe changes in mood, improved confidence, increased bodily awareness, or changes in garment fit. These subjective indications can supplement objective data and help to provide a more complete picture of progress.

Statistics alone do not determine progress. To have a thorough knowledge of your whole trip, it is critical to evaluate numerous metrics and data. Track your success on a regular basis, whether weekly, biweekly, or monthly, and make improvements to your strategy as appropriate.

Finally, remember that development is not necessarily linear. Don't be disheartened if you experience plateaus and swings. Concentrate on the general trend and the good steps you're taking toward your objectives. Stay patient and consistent, and remember to enjoy each milestone along the road.

Adjusting goals as needed to stay motivated and focused

Changing your objectives is a crucial part of remaining motivated and focused on your muscle-building and fat-reduction quest. As you grow and get a better understanding of your body's response, it's critical to review and adapt your goals to keep them tough but realistic. Here are some things to think about while modifying your goals:

Assess Your Progress: Evaluate your progress against your present goals on a regular basis. Consider the metrics and statistics you've been measuring, such as body composition changes, strength increases, and general well-being. If you routinely reach or surpass your objectives, it may be time to establish new, more ambitious ones. If, on the other hand, you frequently fall short, you may need to rethink and change your strategy.

Be Realistic: Consider your existing situation, lifestyle, and any limits or obstacles you may be facing. Make sure your new goals are practical and feasible within the timeframe you've set. Setting too ambitious and difficult-to-attain objectives might lead to dissatisfaction and demotivation. Find the correct balance between pushing yourself outside of your comfort zone and staying within the range of what is possible.

Break It Down: If you're having trouble meeting your initial objectives, consider breaking them down into smaller, more doable milestones. This might help you stay focused and motivated by allowing you to enjoy little victories along the way. Smaller objectives might also help you stay on track and make the required changes.

Timescale: It is critical to be adaptable to your goals' timescale. While having clear timetables is beneficial, work might occasionally take longer than expected. If you discover that you require extra time to meet your objectives, alter the timeframe appropriately. Remember that making steady progress is more essential than meeting an artificial deadline.

Refocus and alter Priorities: As you progress, your priorities or interests may alter. It's totally fine to change your goals to reflect your changing interests and preferences. For example, you may decide that you want to prioritize strength increases over muscle growth, or you may decide that you want to focus on total health and well-being rather than just cosmetic goals. At each level of your journey, align your goals with what actually matters to you.

Seek Professional Help: If you're having trouble adjusting your objectives or determining the proper changes, consider consulting with a skilled fitness professional or coach. They may give vital insights, assist you in setting realistic and individualized objectives, and provide ongoing support and accountability.

Remember that changing your goals does not imply that you are giving up or failing. It's a proactive strategy for keeping your objectives challenging and in line with your existing talents and desires. Keep adaptable, listen to your body, and make modifications as needed to stay motivated, focused, and on track toward your muscle building and fat reduction goals.

The significance of appropriate form and technique

Preventing injuries and maximizing muscle engagement

Injury prevention and muscular engagement are critical components of any strength training program. You may reduce the chance of injury and enhance muscle activation by focusing on appropriate technique, adequate warm-up and cool-down routines, and adding workouts that target particular muscle groups efficiently. Consider the following strategies:

Good Technique: maintain good form and technique throughout all workouts. This ensures that you're using the right muscles while putting the least amount of strain on your joints and other supporting systems. Consider working with a skilled fitness expert who can give assistance and criticism if you're confused about proper form.

Warm-up and stretching: Before each strength training session, prioritize a thorough warm-up program. Dynamic motions that improve blood flow and prepare your muscles for the forthcoming session should be included. Include stretching exercises, especially for the muscles you'll be targeting, to enhance flexibility and range of motion.

Gradual Progression: Do not plunge into large weights or high-intensity workouts without first establishing a strong foundation of strength and stability. Increase the intensity, weight, and complexity of your workouts gradually over time to allow your muscles, joints, and connective tissues to adapt and reduce the chance of overuse problems.

Mind-Muscle Connection: During each exercise, concentrate on creating a strong mind-muscle connection. Pay attention to how the targeted muscle works throughout its complete range of motion. This maximizes muscular activation and guarantees that the desired muscle fibers are successfully stimulated.

Variation and Targeted Exercises: Include a wide range of exercises that target certain muscle groups from a number of angles. This helps to avoid muscular imbalances, guarantees balanced growth, and lowers the danger of overuse problems. Include complex exercises that engage many muscle groups at the same time, as well as isolation exercises that target specific muscles.

Core Stability: Proper mobility and injury prevention require a strong and stable core. In order to improve core strength and stability, incorporate exercises that target your core muscles, such as planks, Russian twists, and deadbugs.

Listen to Your Body: During your workouts, pay attention to any indicators of discomfort, pain, or weariness. If anything doesn't seem right, change the activity, cut back on the weight, or seek expert counsel. Injuries might result from pushing through discomfort or ignoring warning indications.

Rest and Recovery: Allow enough time between sessions for rest and recovery. Adequate rest allows your muscles to recover and develop stronger, lowering your chances of overuse problems. In order to maximize recuperation, incorporate rest days into your training regimen and prioritize excellent sleep.

Cross-Training: To supplement your strength training regimen, use various kinds of exercise, such as aerobic activity and flexibility training. This improves general fitness and mobility, lowering the chance of muscular imbalances and repetitive strain injuries.

Keep in mind that injury avoidance should always be a primary concern. While pushing your limits is necessary for advancement, it should never jeopardize your safety. By using these tactics and emphasizing appropriate technique, warm-up, and recovery, you may reduce the chance of injury while increasing muscle engagement, resulting in more effective and safer strength training sessions.

Effectively engaging the specific muscle groups

Effectively engaging specific muscle groups during strength training is critical for optimizing the benefits of your sessions. Here are some tips to help you improve muscle activation:

Mind-Muscle Connection: During each exercise, concentrate on the muscle you're targeting. Visualize the muscle in action and focus on contracting and squeezing it throughout its complete range of motion. This intentional effort aids in the formation of a strong mind-muscle link and guarantees that the targeted muscle is performing the majority of the work.

Good Form and Technique: Use good form and technique to efficiently isolate and stimulate the target muscle group. Learn the biomechanics of each exercise and perform it with control and precision. This helps to avoid compensatory movements from other muscle groups and directs the effort to the desired muscles.

Slow and controlled movements: Perform exercises with slow and controlled motions, paying attention to both the concentric (muscle contraction) and eccentric (muscle lengthening) phases. Slowing down the tempo increases the duration under strain and gives the target muscles more opportunity to engage and work harder.

Range of Motion: Use a broad range of motion during workouts to properly stimulate the target muscles. This guarantees that you are training the muscle over its entire range of motion and that muscle fiber activation is maximized. When striving for a greater range of motion, however, be careful not to lose good form or compromise joint stability.

Isolation Exercises: Include isolation exercises that target the specific muscle areas you wish to engage. These exercises concentrate on one joint and one muscle group, allowing for more specific targeting and activation. Bicep curls for the biceps, leg extensions for the quadriceps, and lateral raises for the shoulders are other examples.

Compound Exercises: These are exercises that require numerous muscle groups to function in synergy. While they do not isolate individual muscles as well as isolation exercises, they do produce functional strength and general muscular growth. Squats, deadlifts, bench presses, and pull-ups are a few examples.

Pre-Fatigue Techniques: Exercises that isolate the target muscle group should be prioritized early in your session. You guarantee that the muscle is actively engaged by pre-fatiguing it before moving on to complex workouts that activate numerous muscles. For example, before bench presses, execute dumbbell flies to pre-fatigue the chest muscles.

Include Supersets and Drop Sets: Supersets are two workouts performed back-to-back that target the same muscle region. This increases effort and muscle activation. Drop sets include instantly lowering the weight after attaining muscular exhaustion, allowing for continuous muscle activation at a lower load.

Progressive Overload: Keep your muscles challenged by gradually increasing the intensity, weight, or resistance over time. Progressive loading promotes muscular development while also forcing the targeted muscles to adapt and activate more efficiently.

Monitoring and feedback: Pay attention to how your muscles feel during and after each workout. If you don't feel the target muscle working as it should, reconsider your form, technique, and exercise choice. Experiment with different modifications or changes to improve muscle engagement.

Keep in mind that every person's physique is different, and the efficiency of muscle engagement may vary. Listen to your body, make modifications depending on your own experience, and consult with a fitness professional if necessary. You may enhance your ability to engage and activate specific muscle groups during strength training sessions with constant practice and attention to detail.

Seeking guidance from a qualified trainer if necessary

Seeking the advice of a certified trainer is always advised, especially if you are new to strength training or have specific objectives or concerns. A trainer can provide you with individualized advice, analyze your current fitness level, and build a program that is tailored to your specific needs. Here are some of the benefits of contacting a certified trainer:

Proper Form and Technique: A trainer may teach you the proper form and technique for a variety of activities. This is critical for properly working the specific muscle groups while limiting the danger of damage. They may demonstrate exercises and provide feedback to ensure you're doing them safely and efficiently.

Program Design: A trainer may create a personalized program for you based on your objectives, talents, and any special limits or concerns. They may design an organized and progressive program that improves muscle activation, corrects imbalances, and enhances overall strength and conditioning.

Setting and monitoring objectives: A trainer can assist you in developing realistic and quantifiable objectives based on your intended achievements. They may monitor your progress, make modifications as required, and hold you accountable to keep you on track to meet your goals. Assessments and check-ins with a trainer on a regular basis can provide essential feedback and incentive.

Individualized adaptations: Because each person's body is different, a trainer may offer adaptations and alternate routines to meet any physical limits, injuries, or special requirements. They can modify workouts to work around limitations and ensure that you are properly working the targeted muscles while reducing any potential dangers.

Motivation and Support: Throughout your fitness journey, a certified trainer may provide motivation and support. They can offer encouragement, counsel, and assistance in overcoming obstacles or plateaus. Having a trainer by your side may enhance your confidence and keep you motivated to stick to your training schedule.

A trainer can teach you effective warm-up and cool-down routines, educate you on injury prevention measures, and verify that you're utilizing equipment safely. They can also help you recognize yourself during workouts that require assistance, reducing the possibility of mishaps or injuries.

A trainer may expose you to a variety of exercises, techniques, and training methods to keep your workouts interesting and difficult. They can assist you in progressively progressing, ensuring that you constantly exercise your muscles and avoid plateauing in your growth.

Remember that not all trainers are made equal, so pick a competent and experienced expert. Examine certificates from trustworthy organizations, as well as their skills, specialties, and client testimonies. A qualified trainer will emphasize your safety, individual requirements, and general well-being while guiding you through your strength training journey to effective muscle engagement and optimal outcomes.

CHAPTER TWO
CUSTOMIZING YOUR STRENGTH TRAINING ROUTINE

Determining optimal training frequency and duration

Considering recovery capacity and lifestyle factors

It is critical to consider your recovery capabilities and lifestyle considerations when planning a strength training program. Muscle repair, development, and general improvement all rely on recovery. Here are some important considerations:

Rest Days: Include rest days in your training plan to give your muscles time to recuperate and rebuild. Rest days allow your body to adjust to the stress of training and help you avoid overuse problems. Your individual capacity for healing and the level of your exercises will determine the number of rest days you take.

Sleep: Prioritize excellent sleep since it is critical for good recovery. Each night, aim for 7-9 hours of uninterrupted sleep. Your body releases growth hormones during sleep, which help in muscle repair and recovery. Furthermore, getting enough sleep increases energy levels, cognitive function, and general well-being.

Nutrition: Proper nutrition is essential for muscle healing and development. Make sure you're eating a well-balanced diet that includes enough protein to repair and develop muscle tissue. Include enough carbs for energy and healthy fats for optimal health. To help with muscle recovery, stay hydrated and consider taking post-workout meals or snacks that contain a balance of protein and carbs.

Stress Management: Chronic stress might impair your ability to recuperate. Find stress-reduction practices that work for you, such as meditation, deep breathing exercises, yoga, or engaging in hobbies and activities that you like. Stress reduction can improve your body's capacity to recuperate from exercise.

Lifestyle Factors: Consider your lifestyle circumstances that may have an impact on your rehabilitation, such as physical demands from your job, family duties, and other commitments. Examine whether these elements may have an effect on your capacity to recover sufficiently between exercises. Adjust your exercise frequency, intensity, and volume to fit your lifestyle and recuperation requirements.

Recovery Modalities: Explore several rehabilitation treatments that can help with muscle healing and lessen muscular discomfort. Foam rolling, stretching, massage, contrast baths, and the use of rehabilitation aids such as compression sleeves or percussive massagers are examples of these. Experiment with several ways to see which one works best for you.

Listen to Your Body: Pay attention to how your body feels and reacts to exercise. Excessive tiredness, prolonged muscular pain, or a loss in performance may suggest that you require additional recuperation time. Adjust your workout and give your body the rest it requires.

Periodization: Incorporate a periodization approach into your training plan. This entails alternating between higher and lower intensity stages to allow for appropriate recuperation and avoid overtraining. Periodization can assist you in optimizing your development while controlling your recuperation needs.

Time Management: Examine your time obligations and make sure you have adequate time for training and recovery. Maintaining consistency and long-term improvement will be easier if you balance your schedule and prioritize rehabilitation.

Remember that healing is an extremely personal process, and what works for one person may not work for another. Listen to your body, be aware of your recuperation capabilities, and make any modifications to your training schedule. You may enhance your strength training program and achieve long-term growth while keeping a healthy balance in your life by taking your recovery needs and lifestyle considerations into account.

Combining strength training with other types of Exercise

Maintaining a well-rounded fitness regimen and promoting overall health requires balancing strength training with other types of exercise. Here are some things to think about and recommendations for striking the perfect balance:

Determine Your Priorities: Establish your fitness objectives and priorities. If gaining muscle and strength is your primary goal, devote more time and emphasis to strength training. However, if you have additional goals, like cardiovascular endurance, flexibility, or specialized sport-related aims, include exercises that will help you achieve those as well.

Plan Your Schedule: Make a weekly workout routine that includes a combination of strength training and other types of exercise. To achieve an optimum balance, consider the frequency, length, and intensity of each session. Be honest with yourself about how much time you can devote to exercise and prepare appropriately.

Cardiovascular Exercise: To increase cardiovascular health, endurance, and calorie burn, include cardiovascular workouts such as jogging, cycling, swimming, or aerobic courses. Aim for at least 150 minutes of moderate-intensity cardio or 75 minutes of vigorous-intensity cardio each week, as per health standards. These workouts may be spaced out throughout the week or included in your warm-up and cool-down routines on strength training days.

Flexibility and Mobility Training: Stretching, yoga, and mobility activities can help you improve your flexibility, joint range of motion, and general movement quality. These activities can help you avoid injuries, recover faster, and supplement your strength training regimen. Make time for flexibility and mobility exercises, either separately or as part of your warm-up and cool-down routines.

Active Recovery: Implement active recovery days or low-intensity exercises like walking, light cycling, or easy yoga to enhance circulation, help in muscle repair, and give a respite from more strenuous workouts. Active recovery activities can help minimize muscular discomfort, enhance mobility, and keep your exercise program consistent without overtaxing your body.

Sport-Specific Training: Incorporate sport-specific training into your program if you engage in a certain sport or have special fitness objectives relating to a specific activity. Specific drills, conditioning exercises, or technique training may be included to increase your performance in that particular sport or activity.

Pay Attention to Your Body: Pay attention to how your body feels and reacts to various forms of exercise. If you're feeling tired, have chronic muscular pain, or see a drop in performance, it might be an indication that you need to rebalance your strength training and other activities. Allow for adequate healing time and adjust your schedule as needed.

Periodization: Use a periodization technique in your training program to strategically assign distinct phases to focus on certain goals or activities. For example, you can alternate between times of emphasis on strength training and intervals on cardiovascular endurance or flexibility. This enables you to focus on various parts of fitness throughout the year while maintaining overall balance.

Be adaptable and flexible: Recognize that your fitness requirements and objectives may vary over time. Be open to changing your fitness program and discovering new activities that correspond to your changing interests and priorities. Variety and flexibility may help you stay motivated, avoid plateaus, and maintain a well-rounded approach to exercise.

Remember that achieving the correct balance between strength training and other types of exercise is personal. When developing a balanced training plan, keep your objectives, preferences, and physical abilities in mind. Be adaptable, listen to your body, and seek the advice of a fitness professional if necessary to build an activity regimen that meets your needs and maximizes your overall fitness journey.

Personalizing routines based on Preferences and Goals

Individualizing workout routines based on personal tastes and goals is critical for developing a training plan that is pleasant, sustainable, and aligned with your individual goals. Here are some pointers for personalizing your routine to your specific requirements:

Determine Your Goals: Clearly describe your fitness objectives. Are you seeking to gain strength, decrease weight, improve cardiovascular endurance, increase flexibility, or do all of the above? Understanding your goals can help you plan your regimen.

Consider Your Preferences: Consider the sorts of workouts and activities that you love. If weightlifting bores you, try bodyweight exercises or group fitness courses. Incorporate outdoor activities such as hiking, cycling, or running if you enjoy being outside. Choosing activities that you truly like will boost your motivation and compliance with your schedule.

Determine Your Time Availability: Determine how much time you can devote to exercise each day or week. If time is limited, try high-intensity interval training (HIIT) workouts or shorter, more focused sessions. Alternatively, if you have more time, you may schedule longer training sessions or incorporate numerous activities throughout the week.

Customize Training Frequency: Based on your goals, recuperation capabilities, and time availability, choose the best frequency for your exercises. Aim for 2-4 bouts of strength training each week to allow for proper recuperation. If losing weight is a priority, try adopting a combination of strength and cardiovascular activities, aiming for 4-6 sessions per week.

Select Appropriate Exercises: Select exercises that are in line with your aims and interests. Focus on complex movements like squats, deadlifts, bench presses, and rows if you want to increase muscular strength and hypertrophy. Include exercises like jogging, swimming, cycling, or aerobic classes if you want to improve your cardiovascular fitness. Include exercises that will challenge and stimulate your target muscle groups to keep your regimen varied and engaging.

Modify Intensity and Progression: Depending on your fitness level and goals, adjust the intensity of your exercises. As you grow, gradually increase the weight, repetitions, or length of your workouts. To increase variation and difficulty, use tactics like supersets, drop sets, and pyramid sets. To minimize injuries and enhance effectiveness, emphasize appropriate form and technique.

Include Rest and Recovery Days: Schedule rest and recovery days to allow your body to heal and adapt. Muscle repair and development, as well as injury prevention, require recovery. Listen to your body and alter your program appropriately, allowing ample time for relaxation and recuperation.

Introduce Variation: Include diversity in your regimen to avoid boredom and boost overall fitness. To keep things fresh, try different workouts, training methods, or fitness programs. You may also include exercises such as yoga, Pilates, or outdoor sports to push your body in new ways.

Track and Assess Progress: Track and evaluate your progress on a regular basis to stay motivated and make the required modifications. Keep an exercise log or utilize fitness monitoring apps to document your workouts, strength increases, and weight reduction. Assess your progress on a regular basis and make changes to your program as needed to keep pushing yourself and moving toward your objectives.

Pay Attention to Your Body: Pay attention to how your body reacts to various activities and intensities. If you are experiencing discomfort, extreme exhaustion, or a lack of improvement, modify your regimen. Respect your body's limitations and put safety and injury avoidance first.

Remember to enjoy the process and establish a regimen that works for your own interests and goals. You'll be more likely to stay consistent, inspired, and happy with your fitness journey if you personalize your training program. If you're unclear on how to create a personalized program, try speaking with a fitness professional who can offer advice and support tailored to your individual requirements.

Choosing Endomorph-Friendly Exercises

Compound exercises for full-body strength and Calorie burn

Compound exercises are a great way to increase full-body strength, encourage muscular growth, and burn calories more effectively in your training regimen. Compound exercises use many joints and muscle groups, allowing you to activate huge muscle areas while also performing useful motions. Here are some examples of compound workouts that can assist you in achieving these advantages:

Squats: Squats are a basic, complex exercise that focuses on the lower body, specifically the quadriceps, hamstrings, and glutes. They also work the core muscles to maintain stability and balance. Squats can be done with your own bodyweight, dumbbells, barbells, or a squat rack.

Deadlifts: Deadlifts are a complex exercise that primarily targets posterior chain muscles such as the glutes, hamstrings, and lower back. They also work on core strength, upper back strength, and grip strength. Conventional deadlifts, sumo deadlifts, Romanian deadlifts, and trap bar deadlifts are examples of deadlift variants.

Bench Press: A complex exercise that primarily works the chest, shoulders, and triceps It also works the muscles in the back, core, and stabilizers. Bench presses can be done with a barbell, dumbbells, or a bench press machine.

Overhead Press: Also known as the shoulder press, the overhead press works the deltoids, triceps, and upper back muscles. It also works to stabilize the core. Overhead presses can be done with dumbbells, barbells, or a shoulder press machine.

Pull-ups and Rows: Pull-ups and rows are complex workouts that target the back muscles, including the latissimus dorsi, rhomboids, and rear deltoids. They also work the biceps and the core muscles. Pull-ups are done using a pull-up bar, whereas rows are done with dumbbells, barbells, or cable machines.

Lunges: Lunges are a lower-body complex exercise that targets the quadriceps, hamstrings, glutes, and calves. They also work on core stability and balance. Lunges can be done with your own bodyweight, dumbbells, or a barbell.

Clean and Press: A complex workout that includes raising a barbell from the floor to the shoulders and then pressing it overhead. This exercise works on a variety of muscular groups, including the legs, glutes, back, shoulders, and arms. It works the entire body and improves strength and explosiveness.

You may effectively activate numerous muscle groups, boost overall strength, and burn more calories by including these complex exercises in your training program. Begin with appropriate form and technique, then gradually increase the weight or intensity as your strength and skills develop. Warm up properly before beginning complex exercises, and contact a fitness expert if you need assistance with appropriate execution or adaptations according to your fitness level.

Isolation workouts are used to target particular Muscle groups.

In addition to compound exercises, isolation exercises can be added to your training program to target and isolate certain muscle groups. You may concentrate on gaining strength, size, and definition in certain parts of your body with these workouts. Isolation workouts for specific muscle groups include the following:

Bicep Curls: Bicep curls are an individual workout that primarily works the biceps. Bicep curls can be done using dumbbells, barbells, or cable machines. Standing, sitting, and preacher curls are all variations.

Tricep Extensions: Tricep extensions are exercises that isolate the triceps, which are the muscles on the rear of your upper arms. They can be done using dumbbells, barbells, or cable machines. Overhead tricep extensions, tricep kickbacks, and tricep dips are other variations.

Leg Curls: Hamstring curls isolate the muscles on the back of your thighs. They may be done using a leg curl machine or with resistance bands. Lying leg curls and sitting leg curls are two variations.

Leg Extensions: Leg extensions work the quadriceps muscles, which are located on the front of your thighs. They can be done using a leg extension machine. Single-leg extensions and ankle weights are two variations.

Calf Raises: Calf raises isolate the calf muscles, particularly the gastrocnemius and soleus. They may be done using a calf raise machine, dumbbells, or your own bodyweight. Standing calf raises and sitting calf raises are two variations.

Shoulder lateral rises: Shoulder lateral rises work the deltoids, or shoulder muscles. They may be done with dumbbells or resistance bands. Front rises and bent-over lateral raises are two variations.

Chest Flyes: Chest flyes isolate the chest's pectoral muscles. They may be done utilizing dumbbells, cable machines, or a chest fly machine. Chest flies that slope or descend are examples of variations.

Abdominal Crunches: Abdominal crunches isolate the rectus abdominis, or abdominal muscles. They may be done on the ground or with an exercise ball. Reverse crunches and oblique crunches are two variations.

Back Extensions: These exercises work the muscles in the lower back. They may be done using a back extension machine or a stability ball. Hyperextensions and Supermans are examples of variations.

Isolation exercises allow you to directly target certain muscle groups, which helps to enhance muscular balance, symmetry, and overall definition. Compound exercises should still be the core of your training plan since they provide a more complete and functional approach to fitness. Combine isolation and complex movements to build a well-rounded training program that targets both particular muscle groups and overall strength.

Incorporating functional movements for overall fitness

In addition to compound and isolation exercises, including functional movements into your training regimen will help you improve your overall fitness and ability to do daily activities with ease. Functional motions are actions that you do every day, such as bending, lifting, pushing, pulling, and twisting. You improve your strength, flexibility, coordination, and stability by training your body to move functionally. Here are some useful motions that you may incorporate into your workout routine:

Squat to Press: This exercise combines a squat action with an overhead press, working various muscle groups and increasing core stability and coordination.

Medicine Ball Slams: Medicine ball slams include raising a weighted ball above and smashing it to the ground with great power. This exercise promotes power, core strength, and upper-body explosiveness.

Farmer's Carry: The farmer's carry includes walking while holding heavy weights in each hand, such as dumbbells or kettlebells. It puts your grip strength, core stability, and general muscular endurance to the test.

Push-Ups: Push-ups are a traditional functional action that works the chest, shoulders, triceps, and core muscles. They replicate pushing actions that are ubiquitous in daily activity.

Pull-ups: Pull-ups are a great workout for strengthening the back, arms, and core. They imitate tugging motions such as climbing or lifting items.

Lunges with Rotation: To do a lunge with rotation, perform a lunge while turning the torso to the side. This action promotes balance, stability, and rotational strength, all of which are useful for activities such as sports and reaching for things.

Step-ups: These exercises resemble ascending steps and engage the lower body muscles such as the quadriceps, hamstrings, and glutes. They also help to improve balance and coordination.

Plank Variations: Plank variations include front planks, side planks, and plank rotations, which all train the core muscles and develop stability and balance.

Kettlebell Swings: Kettlebell swings incorporate a hip-hinging action pattern and forceful hip extension, targeting the posterior chain muscles such as the glutes, hamstrings, and lower back.

Agility Drills: Including agility drills, such as ladder drills or cone drills, in your workout routine will help you improve your speed, coordination, and footwork.

By including functional exercises in your training program, you may increase your overall fitness level as well as your ability to conduct daily chores. These movements work numerous muscle groups, put your balance and stability to the test, and build functional strength and mobility. To avoid injuries, begin with appropriate form and technique, gradually increasing the intensity or difficulty as you improve, and always listen to your body.

Creating a well-balanced training plan for muscle growth and fat reduction

Dividing exercises for various muscle groups

A typical strategy for strength training is to divide your exercises into separate muscle groups, which allows you to focus on certain portions of your body throughout each session. This method ensures that each muscle group receives sufficient attention and healing time. Here are some common exercise splits to consider:

Upper/Lower Division:

Workout 1: Concentrate on exercises that target upper-body muscles such as the chest, back, shoulders, and arms. **Workout 2:** Focus on movements that target lower-body muscles such as quadriceps, hamstrings, glutes, and calves.

Push/Pull/Split Legs:

Workout 1: Focus on pushing movements for the chest, shoulders, and triceps. **Workout 2:** Focus on pulling movements for the back, biceps, and rear delts. Workout 3: Concentrate on quadriceps, hamstrings, glutes, and calf movements.

Full Body Split (3-4 days per week):

Workout 1: Squats, deadlifts, bench presses, and overhead presses are examples of complex exercises that target numerous muscular groups. **Workout 2:** Include upper-body workouts such as chest, back, shoulders, and arms.

Workout 3: Concentrate on lower-body movements such as quadriceps, hamstrings, glutes, and calves.

Body Part Division:

Workout 1: Concentrate on a single muscle group, such as the chest and triceps.

Workout 2: Focus on a different muscle group, such as the back and biceps.

Workout 3: Focus on a new muscle area, such as the shoulders or the abs.

Workout 4: Focus on another muscle area, such as the legs.

It's important to keep in mind that your training goals, time availability, and personal preferences will all play a role in determining the exact split you choose.

Consider the following suggestions when designing your exercise split:

- Allow enough rest and recuperation time for each muscle group before retargeting it.

- Compound workouts that activate numerous muscle groups should be prioritized for overall strength and functioning.

- To achieve balanced muscular growth, combine complex and isolated workouts. Increase the intensity and volume of your workouts gradually over time to achieve improvement.

- Listen to your body and make the necessary modifications to avoid overtraining and injuries.

- To reduce the chance of injury, remember to warm up properly before each workout and cool down or stretch afterwards. Additionally, if you need assistance establishing a workout split that matches your individual objectives and needs, talk with a fitness expert or personal trainer.

Incorporating resistance Training and Cardiovascular Exercises

It is critical to integrate both weight training and cardiovascular workouts into a well-rounded fitness plan. These two forms of workouts have distinct advantages and complement one another in boosting general health and fitness. Here's how to include both in your training program effectively:

Plan your workouts: Set aside specified days or times for resistance and cardiovascular activities. This ensures that you devote enough time to each sort of exercise and avoid favoring one over the other.

Make resistance training a priority: Begin each workout session with weight-training exercises. This is due to the fact that resistance exercise demands more concentration and energy, especially when lifting heavier weights. It is best to do these workouts when you are fresh and have enough energy reserves.

Choose Compound Exercises: Compound exercises should be prioritized during resistance training sessions. These exercises train numerous muscle groups at the same time and give a thorough workout. Squats, deadlifts, bench presses, rows, and overhead presses are a few examples.

Incorporate Supersets or Circuits: Consider integrating supersets or circuits to save time and boost the cardiovascular component of your weight training session. This is completing one workout after another with little rest in between, keeping your heart rate up and increasing calorie burn.

Add cardio intervals: Include cardio intervals in your resistance training routines to improve cardiovascular fitness. You can achieve this by alternating sets of resistance exercises with brief bursts of high-intensity workouts like jumping jacks, mountain climbers, or burpees.

Distinct Cardio Sessions: In addition to cardio intervals during resistance training, set aside distinct sessions for cardiovascular workouts. Running, cycling, swimming, brisk walking, or utilizing cardio devices like the treadmill or elliptical trainer are examples of such exercises.

Dedicate separate Cardio sessions: Change up your cardio routines to keep things fresh and challenge your body in new ways. In order to obtain the most cardiovascular advantages, combine high-intensity interval training (HIIT) with steady-state cardio.

Mix up Cardio Activities: Determine the frequency and duration of your resistance training and cardiovascular exercises. Your fitness level, goals, and time availability will determine the frequency and length of your resistance training and cardiovascular workouts. The American Heart Association advises aiming for 150 minutes of moderate-intensity cardiovascular activity or 75 minutes of vigorous-intensity exercise each week in addition to at least 2-3 days of weight training per week.

Determine frequency and duration: Allow for enough rest and recovery: enough rest and recovery are required for the best outcomes and injury avoidance. Schedule recovery days in between sessions and avoid days of heavy training on consecutive days. Use these days of rest for mild stretching, mobility exercises, or active rehabilitation activities such as yoga or easy walking.

Listen to your body: Pay attention to how your body reacts to the mix of weight training and cardiovascular activity. Adjust as required, such as by decreasing training volume or intensity if you're feeling overly tired or increasing it if you're not getting the desired results.

To preserve flexibility and prevent muscular imbalances, remember to warm up before each workout, cool down afterward, and stretch on a regular basis. It's always a good idea to work with a fitness professional or personal trainer to create a training plan that's tailored to your unique objectives, talents, and any underlying medical concerns.

Periodization and Progressive Overload for ongoing improvement

Periodization and progressive overload are fundamental ideas in strength training that promote continual progression and prevent plateaus. You may improve your development and get long-term outcomes by progressively increasing the demands placed on your body and intelligently organizing your training cycles. Here's how to use progressive overload and periodization in your training:

Gradual Overload:

Gradually raise the intensity: Keep your muscles challenged by gradually increasing the weight, resistance, or difficulty level of your workouts. This can be accomplished by raising the weight, the number of repetitions, or the intensity of bodyweight workouts.

Concentrate on volume: Change the overall volume of your workout, which is the sum of weight, sets, and repetitions. To enhance muscle development and adaptability, progressively increase overall volume over time.

Maintain good Form and Technique: Maintain proper form and technique during your exercises.

This allows you to target the desired muscle groups while minimizing the danger of harm. Maintain a training log to keep track of your lifts, repetitions, and sets. Tracking your progress helps you objectively measure your development and make any necessary changes to your training regimen.

Periodization:

Implement a Systematic Plan: Break your training down into several periods or cycles, each with a different emphasis. Hypertrophy (muscle development), strength, and power stages are all common.

Vary intensity and volume: Within each phase, adjust the intensity (load) and volume (sets and repetitions) to induce distinct adaptations. During the hypertrophy phase, for example, emphasis is placed on moderate to high repetitions and moderate weights, whereas the strength phase emphasizes fewer repetitions and larger loads.

Allow for recuperation: Plan intervals of reduced intensity or active recovery to allow your body to rest and regenerate. This reduces overtraining and encourages improved performance in the following phases.

Deload weeks: Include deload weeks in your training schedule to lessen the amount and intensity of your exercises. This brief reduction in training stimulus helps your body recuperate, lowering your chance of injury and mental exhaustion.

Periodic Testing and Reassessment: Assess your progress on a regular basis by integrating testing weeks or particular milestones to gauge your strength and performance gains. This enables you to assess the success of your program and make the required changes.

By combining progressive overload and periodization into your training regimen, you develop an organized and methodical approach to muscle adaptation, plateau prevention, and ongoing progression. Remember to listen to your body, make any adjustments to your training program, and allow for enough recuperation and rest to encourage long-term success and reduce the danger of overtraining. If you're unfamiliar with these principles or want assistance, a competent personal trainer or strength and conditioning expert may provide important direction and support.

CHAPTER THREE
COMPOUND EXERCISES FOR TOTAL BODY STRENGTH

Squats: Benefits and Variations

Squats are one of the most efficient and versatile compound exercises for increasing lower-body strength and total functional fitness. They primarily work the muscles in your thighs, hips, and glutes, but they also activate your core and develop overall body stability. Here are several squat advantages and variations:

Squats provide the following advantages:

Lower body strength: Squats are good for developing quadriceps, hamstrings, and gluteal strength. They target these vast muscular groups, assisting you in developing lower-body power and stability.

Functional movement: Squats are very beneficial for daily tasks since they imitate common actions like sitting and standing up. Improving your squat technique has the potential to improve your entire movement mechanics and mobility.

Core engagement: Squats need core stability, which helps build your stomach and back muscles. Maintaining appropriate posture and stability during numerous physical activities requires a strong core.

Increased calorie burn: Squats are a complex exercise that engages many muscular groups at the same time, which increases calorie expenditure. Squats are excellent for weight reduction and fat burning since they lead to a larger calorie burn during and after your workout.

Improved bone density: Squats are a weight-bearing workout that can enhance bone health and help avoid illnesses such as osteoporosis.

Squat variations:

Bodyweight squats: Squats performed without the use of any additional weight They are great for beginners or those looking to improve their squat technique and strength base.

Goblet squats: In goblet squats, you add resistance to the action by holding a kettlebell or dumbbell at chest level. This variant aids in the improvement of posture, balance, and core activation.

Barbell back squats: Squats with a loaded barbell across your upper back This version allows you to lift greater weights and more intensely targets the posterior chain muscles (glutes and hamstrings).

Front squats: Front squats are performed by positioning a barbell in front of your body and resting it on your shoulders. This variant focuses more on quadriceps and core engagement.

Sumo squats: Sumo squats feature a broader stance and toes that point outward. This version focuses more on the inner thighs (adductors) and can help improve hip mobility.

Bulgarian split squats: In this version, you lift one foot behind you while squatting with the other leg. Bulgarian split squats aid in muscular imbalances, single-leg strength, and hip stability.

Overhead squats: Overhead squats are performed by holding a barbell or weight overhead while squatting. This variant puts your core stability, shoulder mobility, and entire body coordination to the test.

It is critical to maintain good form and technique when executing squats. To return to the beginning position, keep your feet shoulder-width apart or slightly wider, maintain a neutral spine, lower your hips back and down as if sitting in a chair, and push through your heels.

Begin with a weight and variation that are appropriate for your current strength and fitness level, gradually graduating to more difficult variations and greater resistance as you acquire strength and confidence. If you're new to squats or have any underlying medical concerns, speak with a fitness expert or personal trainer to guarantee appropriate form and reduce the chance of damage.

Lower body muscular activation and core stability

Engaging the lower body muscles and maintaining core stability are critical for appropriate technique and optimizing the benefits of squats. Here's how to recruit these muscle groups efficiently during squats:

Muscles of the Lower Body:

Quadriceps: Focus on pushing through your heels and working your quadriceps (front thigh muscles) as you drop into the squat. As you return to your starting posture, imagine pushing the floor away.

Hamstrings and Glutes: As you press your hips back and down, engage your hamstrings (back thigh muscles) and glutes (buttocks). This assists you in maintaining balance, stability, and power throughout the squat. Squeeze your glutes at the peak of the exercise to stimulate these muscles even more.

Calves: Squats also utilize your calf muscles, particularly during the push-off phase. To activate the calves, make sure you're pressing through the full foot, including the balls of your feet and toes.

Core Stability Engagement:

Maintain a neutral spine: During the squat to keep your core muscles engaged. Avoid excessively arching or rounding your back.

Engaging your core muscles helps to support your spine and keep it in normal alignment.

Brace your core: Take a deep breath and brace your core muscles by clenching your abdominal muscles as if you were about to be hit in the stomach before descending into the squat. This generates intra-abdominal pressure, which provides stability and support during the action.

Use your core as a stabilizer: Keep your core tight and engaged throughout the squat. This aids in maintaining appropriate posture and prevents excessive torso leaning or tilting. By intentionally activating your lower body muscles and core during squats, you guarantee that you're targeting the right muscle groups and maintaining stability and control throughout the activity. This not only increases the exercise's efficiency but also helps to prevent injuries.

Remember that appropriate form and technique are critical for activating the desired muscle groups while also guaranteeing safety. Consider working with a skilled fitness expert if you're new to squats or want to improve your technique. They can give instructions and feedback to help you activate the proper muscles efficiently.

Deadlifts: Techniques and Variations

Conventional deadlifts, sumo deadlifts, and Romanian deadlifts.

Deadlifts are complex exercises that primarily target the muscles of the posterior chain, such as the hamstrings, glutes, and lower back. There are several deadlift variants, each with its own set of advantages and emphasis on various muscle areas. Here's a rundown of traditional deadlifts, sumo deadlifts, and Romanian deadlifts:

Traditional deadlifts:

Technique: Stand with your feet hip-width apart and your toes pointing forward. Bend your hips and knees while keeping your back straight and your chest elevated. Using an overhand grip, hold the barbell slightly wider than shoulder-width apart. Engage your core, drive through your heels, and extend your hips and knees to raise the barbell off the floor. Keep your spine neutral during the exercise.

Targeted Muscles: Traditional deadlifts typically work the hamstrings, glutes, quadriceps, lower back, and grip strength. As stabilizer muscles, they also involve the core, upper back, and forearms.

Benefits: Deadlifts are a full-body workout that improves general strength and power. They are useful for building posterior chain muscles, increasing hip and knee extension, and strengthening grip strength.

Deadlift Sumo:

Technique: Stand with your feet wider than shoulder width apart and your toes pointing outward at a 45-degree angle. Grip the barbell with your hands inside your legs. Engage your core, drive through your heels, and extend your hips and knees to raise the barbell off the floor. Keep your spine neutral during the exercise.

Muscles Targeted: Sumo deadlifts emphasize the inner thigh (adductor) muscles, glutes, quadriceps, and lower back more than traditional deadlifts. They also work on core strength, upper back strength, and grip strength.

Sumo deadlifts are especially good for people with lengthy torsos or restricted hip mobility. They have a shorter range of motion than traditional deadlifts and can target the inner thigh muscles more efficiently.

Romanian Deadlifts (RDL):

Technique: Standing with your feet hip-width apart and a barbell or dumbbells in front of your thighs, hands facing your body, perform this exercise. Hinge at the hips, letting the weights fall toward the ground while maintaining a straight back and slightly bent knees. Feel the hamstrings squeezing. Reverse the movement by squeezing your glutes at the top and using your hamstrings and glutes to stand up straight.

Muscles Targeted: Romanian deadlifts typically work the hamstrings, glutes, and lower back. They also act as stabilizers by engaging the core.

Benefits: Romanian deadlifts target the posterior chain, namely the hamstrings and glutes. They aid in the improvement of hip hinge mechanics, hip mobility, and hamstring flexibility. RDLs are an excellent exercise for increasing posterior chain strength and stability without putting too much focus on grip strength.

Including these deadlift variants in your strength training regimen can give you a well-rounded approach to addressing posterior chain muscles and increasing overall strength and power. Before progressively increasing the load, it's necessary to start with lighter weights and focus on appropriate form and technique. Consider working with a skilled trainer to gain instruction and feedback if you're new to deadlifts or want to ensure proper execution.

Targeting the posterior chain and building overall strength

Building general strength and targeting the posterior chain is critical for functional mobility, athletic performance, and overall muscle balance. The posterior chain includes the muscles on your behind, such as your hamstrings, glutes, lower back, and upper back. Here are some workouts and ideas for targeting the posterior chain and increasing overall strength:

Deadlift Variations: Traditional deadlifts, sumo deadlifts, and Romanian deadlifts are all effective workouts for targeting the posterior chain. They work the hamstrings, glutes, and lower back, as well as other muscles like the quadriceps and core. Deadlifts increase general strength, power, and muscular mass.

Hip Thrusts: Hip thrusts are excellent for targeting the glutes and strengthening the posterior chain. Sit on the ground with your upper back against a bench, place a barbell or weight across your hips, and raise your hips off the ground. For maximal stimulation, squeeze your glutes at the apex of the exercise.

Glute Bridges: Similar to hip thrusts, glute bridges can be performed without the need for additional weight. Lie on your back, legs bent, feet flat on the ground. Bridge up by lifting your hips off the ground and clenching your glutes. Glute bridges are exercises that serve to engage and develop the glutes, hamstrings, and lower back.

Good Mornings: Good mornings are a complex exercise that works the hamstrings and lower back. Begin by standing hip-width apart with a barbell over your upper back. Maintain a neutral spine by hingeing forward at the hips with a modest bend in your knees. Drive through your hips and engage your hamstrings and glutes to return to the beginning position.

Reverse Lunges: Reverse lunges are an excellent way to work the hamstrings, glutes, and quads. Begin by standing erect and taking a stride backward, dropping your back leg to the ground while maintaining a 90-degree angle with your front knee. To return to the beginning position, push through your front heel. Alter the legs to complete the set.

Kettlebell Swings: Kettlebell swings are a dynamic workout that works the glutes, hamstrings, and core. Holding a kettlebell with both hands, stand with your feet shoulder-width apart. Swing the kettlebell between your legs while hinged at the hips. Extend your hips explosively, swinging the kettlebell up to chest level while keeping a neutral spine. Return the swing between your legs with control.

Back Extensions: Back extensions are an excellent way to address the lower back muscles. To do this exercise, use a back extension bench or a stability ball. Lie face down on the bench or ball with your hips resting on it and your feet anchored. Lift your upper body by contracting your lower back muscles, then slowly lower it back down.

While addressing the posterior chain, appropriate form and technique are critical. Begin with lighter weights and raise the burden gradually as your strength increases. Aim for a well-rounded training regimen that includes workouts for all muscle groups. Consulting with a trained fitness expert may provide individualized coaching and ensure you're successfully and safely addressing the posterior chain.

Bench Press: Proper form and modifications

Flat bench press, incline bench press, and dumbbell variations

The bench press is a well-known compound exercise that works the chest, shoulders, and triceps. There are several bench press varieties that provide distinct advantages and target certain parts of the chest. The flat bench press, incline bench press, and dumbbell variants are as follows:

Bench Press (Flat):

Technique: Lie flat on a seat with your feet firmly planted on the ground. Take an overhand hold on the barbell, a little wider than shoulder-width apart. Lower the barbell to your mid-chest by bending your elbows and keeping them at a 45-degree angle to your torso. Return the barbell to the beginning position by fully extending your arms.

Targeted Muscles: The flat bench press primarily targets the pectoralis major (chest muscles), anterior deltoids (front shoulder muscles), and triceps. It works the core and stabilizer muscles as well.

Benefits: A flat bench press is great for general chest development, strength increases, and increasing upper body pushing power.

Incline Bench Press:

Technique: Adjust the inclination of the bench to 30–45 degrees. Lie back on the bench and take an overhand hold on the barbell, hands slightly wider than shoulder-width apart. Lower the barbell to your upper chest while maintaining a 45-degree angle between your elbows and your torso. Return the barbell to the beginning position by fully extending your arms.

Muscles Targeted: The upper chest (clavicular head of the pectoralis major), front shoulder muscles, and triceps are the primary objectives of the incline bench press. It works the core and stabilizer muscles as well.

Benefits: The inverted bench press develops the upper chest, resulting in a more rounded and developed chest look. It also helps to build up the shoulders and triceps.

Dumbbell Exercises:

Dumbbell Bench Press: Lie flat on a bench with a dumbbell in each hand at shoulder height. Lower the dumbbells to your sides, holding your elbows at a 45-degree angle. Return the dumbbells to their starting position by fully extending your arms.

Incline Dumbbell Bench Press: Similar to the incline bench press, but using dumbbells instead of a barbell. Adjust the bench to the correct inclination angle and replace the barbell with dumbbells.

Dumbbell Flyes: Lie flat on a bench with your palms facing each other, holding a dumbbell in each hand over your chest. Lower the dumbbells in a broad arc out to the sides, experiencing a stretch in your chest. Return the dumbbells to the beginning position while pressing your chest muscles.

Because of the greater demand for balance and control, dumbbell variants of the bench press present an added test for your stabilizer muscles. They also have a wider range of motion than the barbell bench press, which can help engage the chest muscles even more.

It is critical to adopt appropriate form, maintain a solid core, and prevent excessive arching of the lower back when completing any bench press variant. Begin with a weight that allows you to keep proper form and progressively raise the load as your strength increases. Consider working with a certified trainer to master appropriate technique and receive coaching if you are new to these workouts.

Strengthening the Chest, Shoulders, and Triceps

Developing chest, shoulder, and triceps strength is critical for upper body power, stability, and total functional fitness. Here are some workouts that are useful for targeting specific muscle groups:

Chest:

Bench Press with a Barbell: This combination exercise works the chest, shoulders, and triceps. Place your hands slightly wider than shoulder-width apart on a flat bench and hold the barbell. Lower the barbell to your mid-chest, then push it back up to start.

Dumbbell Chest Press: Lie on a flat bench, palms facing forward, with a dumbbell in each hand. Extend your arms directly over your shoulders. Lower the dumbbells to your sides, then push them back up.

Push-ups: Push-ups are a bodyweight workout that works the chest, shoulders, and triceps. Put your hands slightly wider than shoulder-width apart in a plank stance. Lower your body until your chest is almost touching the ground, then push yourself back up.

Shoulders:

Overhead Press: This workout works the triceps and shoulders. Stand with a barbell or dumbbells at your shoulders. Lift the weight until your arms are completely extended, then drop it again.

Sit on a bench with a dumbbell in each hand at shoulder height and perform a dumbbell shoulder press. Dumbbells should be raised until your arms are completely extended, then lowered.

Lateral Raises: Place dumbbells at your sides and lift them until your arms are parallel to the floor. The medial deltoids (side shoulder muscles) are targeted in this workout.

Triceps:

Tricep dips: Place your hands behind you on parallel bars or a stable platform. Bend your elbows to lower your body, then push back up to the starting position.

Close-grasp Bench Press: Lie on a flat bench with your hands shoulder-width apart and grasp the barbell. Lower the barbell to your lower chest and push it back up, keeping your elbows tight to your torso.

Tricep pushdowns: Attach a rope or bar at chest level to a cable machine. Overhand, hold the rope or bar and push it down, completely extending your arms. Concentrate on contracting your triceps.

It is critical to gradually raise the weights and push your muscles over time. To improve strength, aim for 8–12 repetitions per set. Allow enough time between sets and use these exercises in a well-rounded training plan that also incorporates other muscle groups.

Furthermore, a good diet and rest are essential for muscle rehabilitation and development. Make sure you're getting enough protein, healthy fats, and complex carbs to help your muscles grow. To avoid overtraining and injuries, keep your training constant, gradually raise the weights, and listen to your body.

Overhead Press: Strengthening the Upper Body

The overhead press is a fantastic exercise for developing upper-body strength, especially in the shoulders, upper chest, and triceps. It entails lifting weights while standing or sitting. Here's how to do the overhead press and what it can do for you:

Technique:

Stand or sit with your feet shoulder-width apart and an overhand grip on a barbell or dumbbells at shoulder level.

Brace your core, keep your knees slightly bent, and engage your glutes for stability.

By raising your arms straight up, press the weight overhead. Avoid arching your back by keeping your elbows slightly forward.

Once the weight is fully stretched overhead, slowly lower it back to the starting position.

Benefits:

Shoulder and upper chest strength: The overhead press focuses on the deltoid muscles in the shoulders, particularly the anterior deltoids. It also, to a lesser extent, works the upper chest muscles (the clavicular head of the pectoralis major), adding to general upper body strength development.

Triceps Activation: During the overhead press, the triceps act as a synergistic muscle, helping in the pressing movement and adding to arm strength.

Core Stabilization: The overhead press works the core muscles, especially the abdominals and lower back, to keep the action stable and controlled.

Functional Strength: Because the overhead press replicates real-life motions like lifting or pushing items overhead, it is a functional workout that may improve your daily activities.

Consider the following strategies to optimize the benefits of the overhead press and successfully improve upper body strength:

Begin with a weight that allows you to keep perfect form, then progressively raise the load as you gain strength.

Throughout the workout, keep your spine stable and neutral. Avoid excessive lower back arching or upper back overarching.

Maintain correct breathing and core engagement during the activity.

Avoid excessive velocity or swinging by doing the exercise with calm and methodical movements.

To test your muscles from different angles and provide variety to your workout, include overhead pressing variants such as the dumbbell overhead press, sitting overhead press, or push press.

Remember to properly warm up before executing the overhead press and to listen to your body. If you're new to the exercise, consult with a skilled trainer to ensure appropriate form and technique.

Standing overhead presses, sitting dumbbell presses, and push presses are all exercises.

Standing overhead press, seated dumbbell press, and push press are all forms of the overhead press workout that target upper body muscles and aid in strength development. Each practice is summarized below:

Overhead Press Standing:

Holding a barbell or dumbbells at shoulder height with your palms facing forward, stand with your feet hip-width apart.

Brace your core, keep your knees slightly bent, and engage your glutes for stability. By raising your arms straight up, press the weight overhead. Avoid arching your back by keeping your elbows slightly forward.

Once the weight is fully stretched overhead, slowly lower it back to the starting position. The standing overhead press is a complex exercise that focuses on the shoulders (deltoids), triceps, and upper chest. It also works the core muscles to provide stability. Because of the standing position, this exercise provides for increased activation of the stabilizing muscles.

Dumbbell Press While Seated:

Sit on a back-supporting bench with a dumbbell in each hand at shoulder level, palms facing forward.

Maintain a neutral spine by bracing your core. Extend your arms straight up to press the dumbbells above. Avoid arching your back by keeping your elbows slightly forward.

Once the weights are fully stretched overhead, slowly lower them back to the starting position. A version that gives stability and isolates the shoulder muscles is the sitting dumbbell press. Sitting reduces the participation of the lower body, enabling you to concentrate more on the targeted muscles of the shoulders, triceps, and upper chest.

Push and hold:

Begin by standing with your feet hip-width apart and a barbell at shoulder height.

Perform a short dip by bending your knees slightly.

Extend your legs explosively and use the momentum to force the weight aloft. Finish with fully extended arms and elbows locked out.

Return the weight to its initial position with control.

The push press is a dynamic form of the overhead press in which a leg drive is used to produce momentum. When compared to the rigorous overhead press, it allows you to lift greater weights and trains the same muscle groups—shoulders, triceps, and upper chest—but with an emphasis on power and explosiveness.

Including these variants in your workout program may give you diversity and push your muscles in new ways. Choose the variant that best fits your objectives, equipment availability, and personal preferences. It is critical to maintain appropriate form, manage the action, and gradually increase the weight as you advance.

Muscle definition in the shoulders and upper body

Strength training and a good diet are essential for developing shoulder and upper-body muscular definition. Here are some crucial tactics to help you reach your objectives:

Resistance Training in Steps:

Include workouts that target the shoulder muscles particularly, such as overhead presses, lateral lifts, and upright rows. These workouts can help you gain strength and muscle in your shoulders. Compound movements like bench presses, push-ups, and pull-ups that involve numerous upper body muscles, such as the shoulders, chest, and back, should be included. These workouts help build the upper body and define the muscles. Gradually increase the resistance (weight) over time to keep your muscles challenged and stimulated. Aim for a weight that will allow you to perform 8–12 repetitions with excellent technique while still challenging you.

HIIT (High-Intensity Interval Training):

Include HIIT workouts with upper-body movements like burpees, mountain climbers, and kettlebell swings. These workouts work the shoulders and upper body while also encouraging fat loss and calorie expenditure.

HIIT workouts are efficient at burning extra body fat, which can help show upper-body muscle definition.

Concentrate on proper nutrition:

Consume a well-balanced diet that includes enough protein to assist muscle development and repair. 0.8–1 gram of protein per pound of body weight is a good starting point.

Include lean meats, fish, poultry, eggs, dairy products, legumes, whole grains, fruits, and vegetables among your nutrient-dense foods. If you want to lose body fat and gain muscle definition, keep track of your calorie intake and maintain a tiny calorie deficit.

Consistency and Gradual Overload:

When it comes to improving muscle definition, consistency is essential. Maintain a regular exercise program and prioritize strength training and HIIT sessions.

To keep your muscles challenged, gradually increase the intensity, volume, or weights you utilize in your exercises. This is known as progressive overload, and it promotes muscular growth and definition.

Adequate rest and recovery:

Allow enough time for your muscles to heal between sessions. This promotes muscle repair and development.

Aim for 1-2 rest days each week and emphasize enough sleep to aid in the recuperation process. It is important to remember that gaining muscular definition requires time and patience. It is critical to maintain consistency, challenge yourself with your exercises, and nourish your body properly. It's also a good idea to go to a trained fitness professional who can provide you with individualized advice and design a training plan to help you reach your unique objectives.

Rows and pull-ups: upper and lower body development

Pull-ups and rows are great workouts for strengthening the back and upper body. They work on the primary back muscles, including the latissimus dorsi (lats), rhomboids, and trapezius, as well as the biceps and rear deltoids. Each practice is summarized below:

Pull-ups:

Grip an overhead bar with your palms facing away from you and your hands somewhat wider than shoulder width apart (overhand grip). Hang with your arms completely extended, engaging your core, and keeping your knees slightly bent.

Pull yourself up by pressing your shoulder blades together and using your back muscles. Attempt to raise your chin over the bar.

Lower yourself back down slowly while fully extending your arms.

Pull-ups typically work the lats while also engaging the upper back and arms. They are a difficult bodyweight exercise that may be adjusted with the use of support bands or a pull-up machine if necessary.

Rows:

Stand with your feet hip-width apart and an overhand grip on a barbell, dumbbells, or cable connection.
Bend your knees slightly, lean forward at the hips, and maintain a straight back.

Squeeze your shoulder blades together and keep your elbows close to your body to pull the weight towards your torso.

Maintain control throughout the action as you slowly reduce the weight back to the starting position.

Rows may be done with a variety of equipment, including barbells, dumbbells, resistance bands, and cable machines. They work the same muscles as pull-ups, but additionally the biceps and rear deltoids. Row variants such as bent-over rows, single-arm rows, and inverted rows offer varying angles and degrees of difficulty.

Benefits of Pull-ups and Rows for Back and Upper Body Development:

Increased Back Strength: Both exercises target the back muscles, assisting in the development of strength and the improvement of posture.

Upper Body Muscle Definition: Pull-ups and rows activate several upper body muscles, which contribute to general muscular definition in the back, arms, and shoulders.

Grasp Strength: These workouts need a strong grasp, and they can enhance grip strength and forearm growth over time.

Pull-ups and rows simulate real-life pulling actions, making them good for functional strength and everyday tasks.

Consider the following suggestions to get the most out of your pull-ups and rows:

Begin with variations or adaptations that are appropriate for your current fitness level and progressively graduate to more difficult ones. Maintain good form and technique to guarantee adequate muscle engagement and limit injury risk.

Include both exercises in your upper body workouts 1-2 times per week, with appropriate rest and recuperation in between.

If you have trouble with pull-ups, try aided variants or concentrate on developing strength with workouts that target the same muscle areas, such as lat pulldowns or inverted rows. As with any workout, listen to your body, start with suitable weights or adaptations, and progressively increase the intensity as you gain strength. A skilled fitness expert may give further instruction and assist in tailoring your training routine to your unique requirements and goals.

Pull-ups with a wide grip, aided pull-ups, and bent-over rows

Wide-grip pull-ups, assisted pull-ups, and bent-over rows are all good workouts for building upper and lower body strength. Each practice is examined in further detail below:

Pull-ups with wide grips:

Position yourself beneath a pull-up bar with a broad overhand grip that is wider than your shoulders.
Hang from the bar, arms fully extended, and body straight.

Pull your torso upward with your back muscles until your chin clears the bar.

Lower yourself slowly until your arms are completely extended again.

Wide-grip pull-ups primarily target the latissimus dorsi (lats) and work the upper back, shoulders, and arm muscles. The broad grip encourages lat activation and tests your strength and stability.

Pull-ups with a partner:

If you are unable to execute full pull-ups, you can supplement with assistance bands or a pull-up machine.

Adjust the weight on the pull-up machine or secure an aid band around the pull-up bar to an appropriate level.

Repeat the wide-grip pull-up method, focusing on using your back muscles and moving your body higher.

The assistance band or gadget will help you by lessening the strain on your muscles. You may progressively increase strength and proceed to unassisted pull-ups by doing assisted pull-ups. As you gain strength, you may progressively reduce the help or transition to unassisted pull-ups.

Rows with a bent-over position:

Holding a barbell, dumbbells, or kettlebells with an overhand grip, stand with your feet shoulder-width apart.

Bend your knees slightly, lean forward at the hips, and maintain a straight back.

Pull the weight towards your body by pressing your shoulder blades together while your arms are completely extended.

Lower the weight back down slowly while fully extending your arms.

Bent-over rows primarily target the upper back muscles, such as the lats, rhomboids, and rear deltoids. They also work the biceps and lower back. This exercise aids in the improvement of posture, upper-body strength, and muscular definition.

Wide-grip pull-ups, assisted pull-ups, and bent-over rows have the following advantages:

Increased Back Strength: These workouts strengthen and stabilize the back muscles. Improved Posture: Back muscle strengthening helps to improve posture and spinal alignment. **Upper Body Muscle Development:** Wide-grip pull-ups, assisted pull-ups, and bent-over rows work a variety of upper body muscles, including the lats, rhomboids, biceps, and rear deltoids, resulting in better muscle definition. **Core Stability and Engagement:** Pull-ups and bent-over rows both need core stability and engagement, which promote total core strength. Wide-grip pull-ups, aided pull-ups, and bent-over rows can help you attain a well-rounded back and upper body growth by including them in your upper body routines. As you gain strength and proficiency in the exercises, gradually increase the intensity, volume, or weights you utilize.

Remember to emphasize appropriate form and seek the advice of a certified fitness expert if you require assistance or have special concerns.

Strengthening the back, biceps, and overall upper body muscles

It is critical to strengthen the back, biceps, and upper body muscles in order to have a balanced and well-developed physique. Here are some workouts that target certain muscle groups specifically:

Pull-Ups:

Pull-ups should be done with an overhand grip, hands slightly wider than shoulder-width apart. Hang with your arms fully extended from a pull-up bar.

Pull your torso upward with your back muscles until your chin clears the bar.

Lower yourself slowly until your arms are completely extended again.

Pull-ups primarily work the latissimus dorsi (lats), as well as the upper back, biceps, and shoulders.

They are an excellent compound exercise for developing general upper-body strength.

Rows with a bent-over position:

Holding a barbell, dumbbells, or kettlebells with an overhand grip, stand with your feet shoulder-width apart.

Bend your knees slightly and lean forward at the hips while maintaining a straight back.

Pull the weight towards your body by pressing your shoulder blades together while your arms are completely extended.

Lower the weight back down slowly while fully extending your arms.

Bent-over rows work the upper back muscles, including the lats, rhomboids, and rear deltoids, as well as the biceps. They aid in the development of upper-body strength, posture, and general back strength.

Curls on the biceps:

Hold dumbbells or a barbell with an underhand grip and stand with your feet shoulder-width apart.
Keep your elbows close to your sides and your arms completely extended.

Curl the weight upwards towards your shoulders by contracting your biceps.

Slowly return the weight to its initial position.

Bicep curls are exercises that isolate and target the biceps muscles. They aid in the development of biceps strength, size, and definition, adding to overall upper body attractiveness.

Push-Ups:

Begin on a high plank with your hands slightly wider than shoulder-width apart.

Bend your elbows and lower your body to the ground while maintaining your body straight. Return to the beginning posture by pushing through your palms to extend your arms. Push-ups generally work the chest muscles (pectorals), but they also work the triceps, shoulders, and core. They are a type of complex exercise that strengthens the muscles of the upper body.

Overhead Press::

Hold dumbbells or a barbell at shoulder height and stand with your feet shoulder-width apart. By extending your arms and keeping your core engaged, press the weight above.

Return the weight to shoulder height with control.

Overhead presses work the triceps, upper back, and core while targeting the shoulders (deltoids). They help to strengthen the upper body and stabilize the shoulders.

Incorporate these exercises into your upper body training program, aiming for a mix of complex exercises (like pull-ups and bent-over rows) and isolation exercises (like bicep curls). Changing up your sets, repetitions, and weights will aid in muscular growth and development. Maintain appropriate technique and consider working with a competent fitness expert to design a program that is tailored to your specific objectives and fitness level.

CHAPTER FOUR

TARGETED EXERCISES FOR PROBLEM AREAS

Leg Exercises for Building Lean Muscle and Toning

Strength training routines that focus on the main muscle groups in the lower body are necessary to develop lean muscle and tone the legs. The following leg workouts are good for developing lean muscle and toning:

Squats:

Your toes should be turned out slightly when you stand with your feet hip-width apart.

Bend your knees and hips to lower your body as if you were reclining on a chair.

Maintain a raised chest and toe-to-knee alignment. In order to go back to the beginning position, drive through your heels.

Squats work the glutes, hamstrings, and quadriceps, which contribute to the development of total leg strength and muscular definition.

Lunges:

Place your feet hip-width apart as you stand. Your body should be lowered until your front thigh is parallel to the ground by bending both knees while taking a forward step with one leg.

Maintain a raised chest and a straight back. Repeat on the opposite side, pushing through your front heel to go back to the beginning position. In addition to working the hamstrings and calves, lunges primarily work the quadriceps and glutes. They aid in strengthening the legs, enhancing balance, and toning the lower body.

Deadlifts:

While holding a barbell or dumbbells in front of your thighs, stand with your feet hip-width apart. Keep your shoulders back and your back straight as you lean forward at the hips.

Keeping the weight close to your legs, lower it toward the earth.

To raise the weight back up, drive through your heels and tighten your glutes and hamstrings.

In addition to working the lower back and quadriceps, deadlifts primarily work the hamstrings and glutes.

They are a complex exercise that bolsters the posterior chain as a whole.

Step-Ups:

Stand in front of a step or bench.

Step one foot onto the bench and raise your body up by pushing through your heel.

Put your other foot on the bench and come to a full standing position.

Return to the ground and repeat on the opposite side. Step-ups work the glutes, hamstrings, and quadriceps.

They add a cardiovascular element to your leg workout and also train the calves.

Calf Raise:

As you stand with your feet hip-width apart, if necessary, grip a solid support.

Lifting your heels off the ground, stand up on the balls of your feet.

You should feel a stretch in your calves when you bring your heels back down.

The appropriate number of times should be repeated.

Calf raises assist in increasing the strength and definition of the lower legs by focusing particularly on the calf muscles (gastrocnemius and soleus).

Include these leg workouts in your strength training regimen, aiming for two to three weekly sessions. To keep your muscles guessing and to progressively raise the weight as you gain strength, change the number of sets and repetitions. To minimize injuries and increase flexibility, prioritize using perfect technique, warm up before your workout, and stretch afterward.

Leg press variants, split squats, and lunges

Along with the exercises already listed, lunges, split squats, and several varieties of the leg press are other good leg workouts for creating lean muscle and toning. How to carry out these workouts is as follows:

Lunges:
Place your feet hip-width apart as you stand.

Keep your torso upright as you advance on one leg. Bend both knees until your back knee is almost touching the ground or barely there.

To go back to the beginning position, drive through your front heel.

On the opposite leg, repeat the motion. Lunges are a wonderful exercise for developing leg strength and stability since they focus primarily on the quadriceps, hamstrings, and glutes.

Squat Splits:

Place one foot forward on a seat or step as you stand, then place the other foot behind you.

Bend both knees until your back knee is almost touching the ground or barely there. To go back to the beginning position, drive through your front heel.

On the opposite leg, repeat the motion.

The quadriceps, hamstrings, and glutes are worked out during split squats, commonly referred to as static lunges. They aid in enhancing stability, balance, and leg strength.

Variations of the leg press

Leg Press Machine: Place your feet on the footplate of the leg press machine with your legs hip-width apart.

Extend your legs to push the footplate away from your torso.

To bring the footplate back closer to your body, flex your knees.

The appropriate number of times should be repeated.

Single-Leg Press: This workout is similar to the leg press machine, except you only use one leg at a time.

While the other leg is raised or resting on a solid surface, place one foot on the footplate.

Utilizing the working leg, move the footplate away from your body before lowering it again.

Repeat on the other leg after switching.

Leg press variants provide a difficult workout for leg strength and hypertrophy since they target the quadriceps, hamstrings, and glutes. People who might have balance or coordination issues might greatly benefit from these workouts.

Your leg training regimen will be more interesting and effective if you incorporate variants of lunges, split squats, and leg presses. Include these exercises in your workout routine, being sure to pick weights and exercise variants that will allow you to carry out the exercises with good form and control. As your strength develops, gradually raise the resistance. Always pay attention to your body and modify the intensity of your workouts in accordance with your fitness level and goals.

Strengthening the Legs and shaping the Lower Body

Compound exercises and isolation exercises that target the main muscle groups in the legs should be used in conjunction to build leg strength and shape the lower body. The following are some top leg workouts for building strength and toning the lower body:

Squats: As was already noted, squats are a staple leg workout that work the glutes, hamstrings, and quadriceps. They encourage muscular development and aid in increasing total leg strength.

Lunges: Since they work the quadriceps, hamstrings, glutes, and calves, lunges are great for toning the lower body. To engage various muscular areas, you can execute walking lunges, stationary lunges, or reverse lunges.

Step-Ups: The quadriceps, hamstrings, and glutes are the main muscles that step-ups target. Stepping up onto a bench or other raised surface forces your lower body to lift your body weight.

Split squats come in different varieties, such as the Bulgarian split squat. It entails squatting with the front leg while placing one foot behind you on a raised platform, such as a bench. Bulgarian split squats work the glutes, hamstrings, and quadriceps while strengthening and toning the legs.

Leg Press: The leg press machine enables you to use greater loads to target the glutes, hamstrings, and quadriceps. You can efficiently increase your leg strength and muscle definition by pushing against the machine's resistance.

Glute Bridge/Hip Thrust: Although the hamstrings and lower back are also worked during this exercise, the glutes are the primary area of focus. Squeeze your glutes as you lift your hips off the floor while lying on your back with your feet flat on the floor and your knees bent.

Calf raises: To build strength and define the lower legs, calf raises primarily target the calf muscles (gastrocnemius and soleus). They can be carried out on a step or a calf raise machine.

To build leg strength and shape the lower body, keep in mind that consistency and gradual overload are essential. As your strength increases, progressively increase the resistance or weight while performing these exercises two to three times each week. Furthermore, combining strength training with a healthy diet and general calorie restriction can support lower-body muscle definition and fat reduction.

**Core strengthening and definition workouts
Mountain climbers, Russian twists, and Planks**

While not explicitly leg exercises, planks, Russian twists, and mountain climbers are powerful core-engaged motions that can help build general lower body strength and shape by enhancing stability, enhancing calorie burn, and enhancing muscle definition. Let's get deeper into these exercises:

Planks: Planks are an isometric exercise that focuses largely on the core muscles, such as the glutes, lower back, and abdominal muscles. The muscles in the legs, especially the quadriceps, hamstrings, and calves, are also worked during planks, which also emphasize core strength. You may improve general stability and support for lower body motions by strengthening your core.

Russian Twists: The obliques, or the side muscles of the core, are the focus of this dynamic workout. They entail rotating the body from side to side while gripping a weight or maintaining a tight grip on the hands. Even while the lower body's muscles, such as the hip flexors, glutes, and quadriceps, are also engaged during the twisting action, which primarily targets the core, the lower body as a whole gains strength and stability.

Mountain Climbers: This dynamic and challenging workout works the legs, shoulders, chest, and core. They entail getting into a plank posture and alternatively ascending by pushing the knees in toward the chest. Mountain climbers use the lower body muscles, such as the quadriceps, hamstrings, and calves, while also posing a cardiovascular strain. This activity can aid in calorie burning and encourage total lower body muscular tone and definition.

The workouts for building leg strength and shaping the lower body may not include planks, Russian twists, and mountain climbers, but they do add to overall strength, stability, and calorie expenditure. These exercises, together with specific leg workouts, will provide you with a well-rounded approach to accomplishing your fitness objectives. As your level of fitness increases, remember to complete these exercises correctly and progressively increase the intensity and time.

Building core stability and enhancing abdominal definition

Including specialized workouts that target the core muscles is crucial to developing core stability and improving abdominal definition. There are other workouts that concentrate on developing core stability and improving abdominal definition in addition to planks, Russian twists, and mountain climbers.

Bicycle Crunches: Lie on your back with your hands behind your head and perform bicycle crunches by bringing your knees close to your chest. Lift your shoulder blades off the floor, straighten your right leg, and alternate bringing your right elbow to your left knee. Cycle through the opposite side and repeat. The rectus abdominis, obliques, and hip flexors are worked out during bicycle crunches.

Crunches in reverse: Lie on your back and pull your legs off the floor with your knees at a 90-degree angle. Bring your knees up to your chest while using your core to lift your hips off the floor. Repeat by bringing your hips back down gradually. Lower abs are the focus of reverse crunches.

Plank Variations: Plank variants can serve to test and improve the core muscles in addition to the conventional plank. These include side planks, forearm planks, and planks with leg lifts.

Russian Twists with Weight: Sit on the floor with your knees bent and your feet raised off the floor to do a Russian twist with weight. Twist your torso from side to side while holding a weight or medicine ball in front of your chest. Touch the weight to the ground on each side. Russian twists strengthen rotational stability by focusing on the obliques.

Cable Woodchops: Stand close to a cable machine or use a resistance band that is fastened at shoulder level to do cable woodchops. Pulling the cable across your body while maintaining an engaged core requires holding the grip with both hands and rotating your torso diagonally. This exercise strengthens rotational power while focusing on the obliques.

Hanging Leg Raises: Leg raises while hanging with your arms fully extended from a pull-up bar Lift your legs toward your chest while engaging your core, then gently bring them back down. Lower abs and hip flexors are worked during hanging leg lifts.

As you perform these exercises, keep your attention on maintaining appropriate form and control. Start with a weight or amount of resistance that pushes you but still enables you to use proper form. To keep your core muscles challenged, progressively increase the intensity and difficulty of the exercises as you advance. Consistency will aid in revealing the definition in your abdominal muscles over time, combined with a balanced diet and general calorie control.

Arm and shoulder exercises for improved tone and definition

Shoulder presses, Tricep dips, and Bicep curls

The arm and shoulder muscles may be worked using bicep curls, tricep dips, and shoulder presses. The advantages of each workout are broken down below:

Bicep curls: The bicep muscles on the front of the upper arm are the main target of bicep curls. Resistance bands, dumbbells, or barbells can all be used to carry out these exercises. With your palms facing forward and your elbows close to your sides, stand holding a weight in each hand. Keep your upper arms steady and curl the weights up toward your shoulders. Controlled weight reduction of the lifted objects. Bicep curls contribute to bicep strength and definition.

Tricep Dips: The triceps, which are found on the back of the upper arm, are the main focus of tricep dips. Tricep dips can be done on a bench or parallel bars. Fingers pointing forward, place your hands first on the bars or the edge of the bench. When your upper arms are parallel to the ground, lower your body by bending your elbows while keeping them close to your body. Return to the beginning posture by pushing yourself up. The triceps are made stronger and more toned with tricep dips.

Shoulder Presses: Also referred to as overhead presses, shoulder presses work the shoulders' deltoid muscles. They can be carried out with the use of barbells, dumbbells, or a shoulder press machine. With the palms facing forward, place the weights at shoulder height to begin. Once your arms are completely extended and the weights are overhead, bring them back down to shoulder height. Shoulder presses aid in deltoids muscle definition and shoulder strength development.

It's crucial to maintain good form and technique when carrying out these workouts. Use weights that will allow you to control the exercise properly and perform the necessary number of repetitions. Increase the weight gradually as your strength increases. A variety of rep ranges, including higher reps for muscular endurance and lower reps for muscle strength, can also be included to maximize outcomes.

It's also important to note that although these workouts focus on particular muscle groups, they also work other muscles as stabilizers or synergists. Make sure you have a well-rounded fitness program with activities that target different muscle groups and permit enough time for rest and recuperation.

Sculpting and toning the arms and shoulders

Combining strength workouts with aerobic training can be useful for shaping and toning the arms and shoulders. Here are some techniques and activities to focus on these areas:

Resistance Exercises:

A. **Bicep curls:** To target the biceps and encourage arm definition, perform bicep curls with dumbbells, barbells, or resistance bands.

B. **Tricep Dips:** Tricep dips work the triceps and tone the back of the arms by using parallel bars or a bench.

C. **Shoulder Press:** To target the deltoid muscles and chisel the shoulders, perform overhead shoulder presses with dumbbells or a barbell.

D. **Lateral Raises:** These exercises, which target the deltoids and aid in developing shoulder definition, can be done with light dumbbells or resistance bands.

E. Push-Ups: Include push-ups in your regimen to tone and strengthen your upper body while working your chest, triceps, and shoulders.

Exercise Circuits:

Make a circuit-style workout that mixes aerobic activities with resistance exercises for the arms and shoulders. This strategy enhances cardiovascular health, increases general muscular tone, and burns calories. Take bicep curls as an example, then jump jacks or high knees, then tricep dips and mountain climbers, and so on.

High-Intensity Interval Training (HIIT):

Include exercises that engage your arms and shoulders as part of your HIIT routines. Exercise is performed in short, intensive bursts with little rest in between, which promotes fat loss and lean muscle growth. Include exercises that stress your cardiovascular system while also working your upper body, such as burpees, kettlebell swings, and squat thrusters.

Heart-Healthy Exercise:

Include cardiovascular activities like swimming, rowing, boxing, or utilizing an elliptical machine with moving grips that work the arms and shoulders.

These exercises aid in enhancing general muscle tone, calorie burning, and cardiovascular health.

Optimal Nutrition

Keep in mind that a good diet is also necessary for shaping and toning the shoulders and arms. Eat a variety of fruits and vegetables, lean proteins, healthy fats, and whole grains as part of a balanced diet. A sufficient protein intake promotes muscle growth and repair, and calorie intake generally helps with fat reduction and overall muscle definition.

Keep in mind to modify the weight, reps, and intensity depending on your level of fitness and to advance progressively over time. In order to get the results you want, consistency, appropriate form, and patience are essential.

CHAPTER FIVE

MAXIMIZING METABOLISM AND FAT LOSS

Incorporating High-Intensity Interval Training (HIIT)

HIIT benefits for boosting Metabolism and burning Calories

The practice of high-intensity interval training (HIIT) has a number of advantages for increasing metabolism and calorie expenditure. Here is a summary of how HIIT might be beneficial:

Increased Caloric Expenditure: HIIT incorporates short bursts of intensive activity followed by quick rest intervals, increasing caloric expenditure. Your body experiences an increased energy expenditure during and after this form of training. Due to the intensive nature of the intervals, HIIT workouts might result in a greater calorie burn than steady-state cardio routines.

EPOC Effect: Excess Post-Exercise Oxygen Consumption, commonly referred to as the "afterburn effect," is the increased rate of oxygen consumption after physical activity. It has been demonstrated that HIIT produces a larger EPOC impact than steady-state cardio. This implies that even after your HIIT workout is completed, your body continues to burn calories at a high rate in order to replenish oxygen levels and repair muscles throughout the recovery time.

Increased Metabolic Rate: It has been shown that HIIT increases metabolic rate not just when exercising but also for several hours afterward. Due to HIIT's intensive nature, the body's metabolism is stimulated, resulting in a faster metabolic rate throughout the day. The higher calorie burn from this may help with weight reduction or weight management.

Muscle Preservation: Traditional steady-state aerobic activities can cause muscle loss in addition to fat loss, particularly when performed in excess. While largely focusing on fat storage, HIIT has been demonstrated to help maintain muscular mass. You may encourage fat loss while preserving or even increasing your lean muscle mass by doing high-intensity interval training, which can also support a greater metabolic rate.

Efficiency in terms of time: When compared to longer cardio sessions, HIIT exercises are often shorter in length. You may burn more calories and have equivalent or even higher cardiovascular benefits with HIIT in less time. This makes HIIT an appealing choice for people with hectic schedules who want to enhance the effectiveness of their workouts.

While HIIT can be very successful in increasing metabolism and burning calories, it can also be very strenuous and may not be right for everyone. It's crucial to start slowly and advance at a rate suitable for your level of fitness. Before beginning any new workout regimen, speak with a healthcare or fitness expert, especially if you have any underlying medical issues.

Including HIIT workouts in your fitness regimen, along with healthy eating habits and other types of exercise, may help you take a well-rounded approach to improving your metabolism, losing weight, and maintaining overall health.

Sample HIIT workouts and intervals for Endomorphs

Here are some illustrations of HIIT exercises and intervals that are appropriate for endomorphs:

Workout 1: Cardio HIIT Circuit

Equipment needed: None

Warm-up: 5 minutes of light jogging or jumping jacks.

Perform each exercise for 30 seconds, followed by 15 seconds of rest. Complete 3 rounds.

a. High Knees

b. Burpees

c. Mountain Climbers

d. Jump Squats

e. Skaters

f. Bicycle Crunches

g. Plank Jacks

h. Jumping Lunges

i. Russian Twists

j. Rest for 1 minute between rounds.

Cool-down: 5 minutes of stretching exercises, focusing on the major muscle groups.

Workout 2: Strength and Cardio HIIT

Equipment needed: Dumbbells, exercise mat

Warm-up: 5 minutes of light cardio, such as jogging or jumping jacks.

Perform each exercise for 40 seconds, followed by 20 seconds of rest. Complete 4 rounds.

a. Dumbbell Squat to Shoulder Press

b. Plank Jacks

c. Dumbbell Alternating Reverse Lunges

d. Mountain Climbers

e. Dumbbell Bent-Over Rows

f. Jumping Jacks

g. Dumbbell Push-ups

h. High Knees

i. Rest for 1 minute between rounds.

Cool-down: 5 minutes of static stretching for the major muscle groups.

Interval Structure:

For both workouts, the intervals follow a 2:1 work-to-rest ratio. This means that you work for a specific amount of time (e.g., 30 seconds or 40 seconds) and then rest for half that time (e.g., 15 seconds or 20 seconds). This interval structure allows for high-intensity efforts followed by brief recovery periods.

Level of Intensity:

Your degree of fitness will determine how intense the workouts are. If you're just getting started, you might need to alter the workouts or shorten the periods. As you advance, progressively increase the intensity by adding weights, extending the intervals, or cutting back on the rest times.

Always pay attention to your body's signals, drink enough water, and keep your form correct when exercising. Before beginning a new workout regimen, it's always a good idea to speak with a fitness expert, especially if you have any underlying health issues or concerns.

Note: These exercises are offered as illustrative examples only. You are welcome to alter them to suit your tastes, the equipment that is available, and your degree of fitness.

Cardiovascular Exercises for Endomorphs

Selecting cardio workouts based on personal interests

To achieve long-term commitment and enjoyment, it's crucial to take individual tastes into account while selecting aerobic exercises.

When choosing aerobic workouts that fit your tastes, take into account the following factors:

Personal Interests: Take into account pursuits that you actually find enjoyable or interesting. If you prefer to dance, for instance, you may choose a dance-based exercise program like Zumba or hip-hop cardio. Running, cycling, and hiking could be more enticing to you if you enjoy being outside.

Variety: Recognize that there are several cardio activities to choose from. Boredom may be avoided and motivation can be maintained by changing up your daily routine with a range of activities. You may attempt sports like basketball or tennis as well as exercises like swimming, kickboxing, jumping rope, and rowing.

Impact on Joints: Think about workouts that are easy on the joints, including cycling, swimming, elliptical training, or utilizing a rowing machine, if you have joint problems or prefer low-impact sports. These sports can provide you with a heart-healthy workout without putting too much strain on your joints.

Accessibility: Take into account how accessible certain activities are. Exercises that require little to no equipment, such as bodyweight exercises, jumping rope, or following along with internet workout videos, are options if you want to work out at home. On the other hand, if you like working out in a gym, you may experiment with the cardio equipment on hand, such as the treadmill, stationary bike, and stair climber.

Social Engagement: For some people, working out with others is both motivating and enjoyable. If you want a social component to your exercise, think about participating in team sports, group fitness courses, or joining a running or cycling club. Your workouts will be more pleasurable as a result of the sense of accountability and camaraderie that this may bring.

Fitness Objectives: When selecting cardio exercises, keep your fitness objectives in mind. Running or cycling are two examples of exercises that may be more suitable if your objective is to increase your cardiovascular and endurance capacity. You might use circuit training or high-intensity interval training (HIIT) workouts if you want to combine cardio with strength training.

Keep in mind that the finest aerobic exercise is the one you will do frequently and that you will love. Start at a comfortable intensity, pay attention to your body, and gradually increase the length or rigor of your exercises over time. It's also advantageous to speak with a fitness expert who can advise you depending on your unique requirements and objectives.

Balancing Cardio with Strength Training for Optimal results

The secret to attaining the best outcomes in terms of general fitness and body composition is to balance cardio with strength training. Following are some pointers to assist you in finding a balance between the two:

Clarify your objectives: Specify your precise objectives. Your training focus may be more strength-oriented with mild cardio workouts if your primary goals are to increase muscle and strength, with some cardiovascular fitness as a secondary objective. A more balanced strategy between cardio and strength training may be appropriate if your goals are overall fitness and weight loss.

Plan Your Training Schedule: Plan your training schedule and set aside particular days or times for both strength and aerobic exercises. This will guarantee that you're giving both forms of exercise the proper amount of attention. For instance, you may commit three to four times a week to strength training and two to three times a week to cardio, with one or two rest days in between.

Prioritize Intensity and Progression: When weightlifting, concentrate on progressive loading by progressively upping the weight, the number of reps, or the difficulty of your workouts over time. This promotes muscle gain and strength. In order to test your cardiovascular system, focus on intensity throughout your cardio workouts. To increase calorie burning and cardiovascular advantages, use intervals, when you alternate between times of high effort and recuperation.

Combine Both in One Session: Combining the two in one session is an option if you're short on time. You may include some cardio in your strength training workouts. For instance, include supersets or circuit-style workouts that alternate brief bursts of aerobic activity like jumping jacks or burpees with weight training. In this manner, you may efficiently complete both tasks in a single session.

Think about timing and sequence: Your performance and energy levels may be affected by the timing and sequence of your aerobic and strength exercises. To ensure that you have enough stamina to lift weights and maintain perfect technique, it is often advised to prioritize strength training before cardio. To find out which order suits you and your body's reaction, you can try out many variations.

Allow for recuperation: Both strength training and cardiovascular activity require enough recuperation. Make sure to include rest days in your training plan so that your muscles have time to recover and adapt. Avoid overtraining since it might impede your development and raise the possibility of injury.

Listen to Your Body: Pay attention to how your body reacts to a combination of aerobic and strength exercise by keeping a close eye on it. Adjust the amount or intensity of your workouts if you feel overly exhausted or see symptoms of overtraining. Finding a balance that meets your specific demands and promotes sustained growth is essential.

Keep in mind that the ideal ratio of cardio to strength training might change depending on a person's objectives, preferences, and physical condition. It's always a good idea to speak with a fitness expert or trainer who can offer tailored advice and assist in creating a comprehensive program that supports your objectives.

Combining Aerobic and strength training for the best outcomes.

Supersets and circuit training for effective workouts

Supersets and circuit training are well-liked exercise methods that may help you work out more effectively and get the most out of your gym time. An outline of these techniques' functions and advantages is given below:

1. Circuit Training: In circuit training, a number of exercises are performed one after the other with little rest in between. Each exercise targets a distinct muscle group or movement pattern. Here is an example of a circuit training workout's structure:

- Choose a series of exercises that concentrate on certain muscle groups or motions.
- Each exercise should be done a certain number of times or for a specified period of time.
- Without stopping, proceed from one exercise to the next until the full circuit has been done.

- If necessary, take a brief break (30–60 seconds) in between circuits.
- For the appropriate number of rounds, repeat the circuit.

There are various advantages to circuit training, including:

Time effectiveness: By completing exercises one after the other, you may engage more muscle groups and increase your heart rate in less time. Increased Calorie Burn: A circuit workout that combines aerobic and strength workouts can increase your calorie burn both during and after the workout.

Improved Cardiovascular Fitness: By keeping your heart rate up throughout the workout, circuit training puts your cardiovascular system to the test.

Muscle Endurance: The circuit training method's continual nature can increase your body's capacity for sustained physical activity.

2. Supersets:

Supersets are combinations of two workouts that often target opposing muscle groups or other body parts. Following are some tips for including supersets in your workout:

- Choose two workouts that target two distinct muscle groups or regions.
- Without a break, perform the first exercise and then the second exercise straight after.

- After doing both exercises, take a brief break (30–60 seconds).
- For the necessary number of rounds, do the superset again.

Supersets have various advantages, such as:

Increased Intensity: Doing workouts back-to-back without recovery puts more strain on your muscles, which can result in an improvement in strength and muscular development.

Time Efficiency: By combining workouts, you may effectively target numerous muscle areas in less time.

Fatigue and Muscle Pump: Supersets can increase metabolic demand and muscle pump, which helps with muscle development and calorie burning.

Supersets can provide your muscles with new stimulation, helping you overcome plateaus and keep your exercises interesting.

Variety and Overcoming Plateaus:

You may reduce the amount of time you spend working out, boost the intensity, and efficiently target numerous muscle groups by including circuit training and supersets into your regimen.

But it's crucial to pay attention to your body, keep good form, and modify the volume and intensity in accordance with your fitness level and objectives. If you need assistance creating a circuit training or superset program that fits your unique requirements, speak with a fitness expert or trainer.

Strategies for maximizing fat loss while preserving muscle mass

It's crucial to have a complete approach that incorporates good nutrition, exercise, and lifestyle choices in order to maximize fat reduction while protecting muscle mass. Here are some practical tactics to support you in achieving this objective:

Moderate Calorie Deficit: Consume a small number of calories less than what your body requires to maintain itself. Aim for a 500–750 calorie deficit per day to help you lose fat steadily while preserving muscle mass.

High-Protein Diet: Consume enough high-quality protein to help muscles recover and be preserved. Per pound of body weight per day, aim for 0.7–1 grams of protein. Lean meats, chicken, fish, eggs, dairy products, lentils, and tofu are all excellent sources.

Resistance Training: Prioritize resistance exercise to preserve and increase your muscular mass. Concentrate on complex exercises that work numerous muscular groups and gradually stress your muscles by upping the weight, the number of sets, or the number of reps. This will encourage fat reduction while preserving muscle.

Incorporate Cardio: Increase calorie burning and improve cardiovascular health by including cardio activities. Select HIIT and moderate-intensity steady-state cardio exercises (such as brisk walking or cycling). Since HIIT encourages calorie burn both during and after exercise, it is highly helpful for fat loss.

Monitor Macros: Keep an eye on your macronutrient distribution while you monitor your macros. To boost overall energy levels, hormone synthesis, and nutrition absorption, provide a proper diet of healthy fats and carbs in addition to enough protein. Depending on your unique demands and preferences, balance your intake.

Prioritize Nutrient-Dense Foods: To maintain your general health and supply necessary vitamins, minerals, and antioxidants, concentrate on complete, nutrient-dense meals. Eat a diet rich in whole grains, lean proteins, fruits, vegetables, and healthy fats.

Manage your Stress and Sleep: Stress and insufficient sleep can impede muscle preservation and fat reduction. Give excellent sleep a high priority to aid in healing and hormone control. Use stress-reduction strategies like deep breathing exercises, meditation, or engaging in activities you like.

Keep hydrated: To assist your metabolism, energy levels, and general health, drink lots of water throughout the day. Water also helps with digestion and controlling hunger.

Track Progress and Adjust: Monitor your progress on a regular basis by keeping note of your measurements, weight, and changes in your body's composition. To keep moving toward your goals, make the necessary adjustments to your diet and exercise routine.

Seek Professional Guidance: Consider working with a licensed nutritionist or a certified personal trainer who can offer you individualized advice and assistance to make the most of your path toward fat loss and muscle maintenance.

Keep in mind that it takes time and consistency to lose fat in a sustainable manner while maintaining muscular mass. Prioritize general health and well-being throughout the process and place a focus on slow, steady improvement.

CHAPTER SIX

NUTRITION AND SUPPLEMENTATION FOR ENDOMORPHS

Importance of a Balanced Diet for Muscle Growth and Fat Loss

A well-balanced diet is essential for both muscle building and fat removal. It supplies the nutrition, energy, and building blocks required for healthy body composition modifications. Here are the main reasons why a balanced diet is essential for muscle building and fat loss:

Meeting Nutrient needs: A well-balanced diet ensures that you are getting a proper number of key nutrients such as proteins, carbs, fats, vitamins, and minerals. These nutrients are essential for a variety of physiological activities, including muscle regeneration, energy production, and general health.

Muscle repair and Protein Synthesis: Protein is required for muscle development and repair. Consuming enough high-quality protein promotes protein synthesis, the process by which new muscle tissue is formed. It also improves the repair of muscular injuries caused by exercise. Lean meats, poultry, fish, dairy products, legumes, and plant-based protein sources can help with muscle development and repair.

Workout Energy: Carbohydrates are the body's major source of energy. They provide you with the energy you need for rigorous exercises and resistance training sessions, allowing you to perform at your peak. Incorporating complex carbs into your diet, such as whole grains, fruits, vegetables, and legumes, guarantees a consistent source of energy for effective exercise and muscular building.

Fat Loss and Energy Balance: Fat loss necessitates a caloric deficit, which means consuming fewer calories than you burn. A well-balanced diet can assist you in creating this shortfall while also delivering the required nutrients. You can manage your energy consumption while still achieving your nutritional needs by incorporating nutrient-dense, low-calorie meals. Balancing macronutrients, such as getting enough protein and healthy fats, can help you feel full and retain muscle mass while lowering your overall calorie consumption.

Micronutrient Support: A balanced diet provides critical vitamins and minerals that promote healthy metabolism, hormone function, and general health. Micronutrients such as vitamin D, calcium, iron, and magnesium are essential for muscular function, bone health, and recuperation.

Sustained Energy Levels: Eating a range of nutrient-dense foods throughout the day gives a constant flow of energy. This contributes to steady blood sugar levels, constant energy levels, and the prevention of energy crashes, which can impair workout performance.

Overall Health and well-being: A balanced diet promotes overall health, which is necessary for long-term muscle growth and fat loss objectives. It supports a healthy immune system, organ function, and hormone levels. When your body is in good working order, you may engage in regular exercise, recuperate from exercise, and maintain a healthy lifestyle.

Individual demands may differ depending on characteristics such as age, gender, exercise level, and special goals. To modify your nutrition plan and ensure it corresponds with your unique requirements and preferences, talk with a certified dietitian or healthcare expert.

Caloric intake, Macronutrient Ratios, and Portion Control.

Caloric intake, macronutrient ratios, and portion management are all significant aspects of gaining muscle and losing fat. Let's look at each of these points individually:

Caloric intake: The total quantity of calories consumed in a day is referred to as calorie intake. To lose fat, you must generate a caloric deficit by eating fewer calories than you burn. This shortfall forces your body to use stored fat for energy. You may need to consume a modest calorie surplus to provide the essential energy for muscle development when building muscle. Individual factors such as exercise level, body composition, and objectives will influence calorie consumption.

Macronutrient ratios: Macronutrients are the three primary energy-producing nutrients: carbs, proteins, and fats. Individual tastes and demands can influence the appropriate macronutrient ratios for muscle building and fat reduction. A basic rule of thumb is to consume more protein to assist muscle development and repair, moderate quantities of healthy fats for hormone synthesis and overall health, and an adequate quantity of carbs to fuel exercise and give energy.

Protein: A sufficient protein intake is essential for muscle development and repair. Consume around 0.7–1 gram of protein per pound of body weight each day. Lean meats, poultry, fish, dairy products, legumes, and plant-based protein sources like tofu and tempeh are all good sources.

Carbohydrates: Complex carbs, such as whole grains, fruits, vegetables, and legumes, should be consumed. These give prolonged energy as well as essential nutrients. Carbohydrate consumption should be adjusted based on exercise level and personal preferences.

Fats: Healthy fats may be found in nuts, seeds, avocados, olive oil, and fatty seafood. These supply vital fatty acids and aid in the generation of hormones. Because fats are high in calories, watch your portion sizes.

Portion Control: Portion control entails regulating the amount of food you consume at each meal and snack. It keeps you from overeating and allows you to better regulate your calorie intake. You may regulate quantities by using smaller plates, weighing food with kitchen scales or measuring cups, and being aware of portion sizes while dining out.

Incorporate a variety of nutrient-dense foods into your meals, including lean proteins, whole grains, fruits, vegetables, and healthy fats.

To avoid overeating, pay attention to hunger and fullness signs. Eat till you're full but not stuffed. High-calorie meals and beverages should be consumed in moderation.

It's crucial to remember that everyone's demands and tastes are different. Exercise level, metabolism, and body composition are just a few examples of the variables that can affect specific recommendations for calorie intake, macronutrient ratios, and portion sizes. A trained dietitian or nutritionist can assist you in personalizing your nutrition plan and optimizing your muscle-building and fat-reduction journey.

They may provide you with advice that is tailored to your personal needs, taking into account any underlying health concerns or dietary limitations.

Lean proteins, complex carbs, and healthy fats are all included.

In order to stimulate muscle building and fat reduction, you must consume lean proteins, complex carbs, and healthy fats. These macronutrients supply the building blocks, energy, and nutrition required for healthy body composition modifications. Here's how to add them to your diet:

Lean proteins:

Choose skinless poultry, lean cuts of meat, fish, eggs, low-fat dairy products, legumes (beans, lentils, chickpeas), and plant-based protein sources like tofu and tempeh as lean protein sources.

Protein should be included in all of your meals and snacks to enhance muscle protein synthesis and help in muscle repair and recovery.

Carbohydrates that are complex:

Choose whole grains over refined grains, such as brown rice, quinoa, whole wheat bread, and whole wheat pasta. These are high in fiber and give long-lasting energy.

Consume a variety of fruits and vegetables since they are high in vitamins, minerals, and antioxidants. These also include important fibers for digestion and satiety.

Legumes and beans are high in complex carbs and protein.

Healthy fats:

Avocados, nuts, seeds (chia seeds, flaxseeds), olive oil, coconut oil, and fatty fish (salmon, mackerel, and sardines) are all good sources of healthy fats.

Because fats are high in calories, watch your portion sizes. Strive for balance and moderation.

Anti-inflammatory omega-3 fatty acids, found in fatty fish, flaxseeds, and chia seeds, can help with general health.

Here are some meal and snack suggestions that include these macronutrients:

Grilled chicken breast with roasted veggies and quinoa on the side

Salmon with steamed broccoli and a sweet potato
Greek yogurt with berries and almonds sprinkled on top

Avocado on whole wheat bread with a cooked egg
Tofu stir-fry with mixed veggies and brown rice
Salad with spinach, grilled chicken, cherry tomatoes, cucumber, and an olive oil dressing
Cottage cheese with fruit slices and a handful of nuts

Remember to alter portion sizes according to your calorie needs and objectives. It's also critical to pay attention to your body's hunger and fullness cues to ensure you're fueling properly and not overeating. Working with a qualified dietitian or nutritionist can assist you in developing a tailored food plan that suits your individual needs and tastes while promoting muscle building and fat reduction.

Macronutrient Ratios and Portion Management

Finding the optimal protein, carbohydrate, and fat ratio

Finding the appropriate protein, carbohydrate, and fat balance is critical for muscle building and fat reduction. Here are some general suggestions to follow in order to obtain a balanced macronutrient intake:

1. Protein:

Aim for high-quality protein sources at each meal. Lean meats, poultry, fish, eggs, dairy products, legumes, and plant-based protein sources like tofu and tempeh are examples.

To boost muscle protein synthesis and improve muscle repair and development, distribute your protein intake equally throughout the day.

Determine your protein requirements depending on your body weight and degree of activity. 0.7–1 gram of protein per pound of body weight per day is a good target.

2. Carbohydrates:

Consume complex carbs such as whole grains, fruits, vegetables, and legumes.

Choose fiber-rich carbs with a lower glycemic

index to give sustained energy and encourage feelings of fullness.

Your carbohydrate intake should be adjusted based on your exercise level and goals. On training days, you may require more carbs to power your exercises, but on rest days, you can cut your consumption significantly.

3. Fats:

Consume healthy fats from foods such as nuts, seeds, avocados, olive oil, and fatty seafood. Aim for a fat balance that includes monounsaturated and polyunsaturated fats (omega-3 and omega-6 fatty acids). When ingesting fats, keep in mind that they are high in calories. Moderation is essential.

4. Individualization:

Because everyone's macronutrient requirements and tolerances differ, it's critical to listen to your body and make modifications as needed. Experiment with various macronutrient ratios and see how your body reacts. Some people may feel better with a little more carbohydrate consumption, while others may thrive with a lower carbohydrate intake.

Consider your level of activity, exercise intensity, body composition objectives, and any nutritional preferences or limits.

Remember that reaching a balanced macronutrient intake is a trial-and-error process. It's critical to examine how your body reacts to various ratios and make modifications based on your own requirements and goals. A trained dietitian or nutritionist may give individualized advice and assist you in determining the ideal protein, carbohydrate, and fat balance for your unique condition.

Monitoring portion sizes to properly regulate calorie intake

Portion control is an excellent approach for controlling calorie consumption and maintaining a healthy diet. Here are some pointers to help you monitor and manage your portion sizes:

Use measurement tools: When you're just starting out, use measuring cups, spoons, or a kitchen scale to correctly measure out servings of food. This might assist you in being aware of proper portion quantities.

Pay attention to serving sizes on food labels: when reading food labels. These labels provide the suggested serving size as well as the number of servings per container. When portioning your meal, use this as a reference.

Visual Cues: When you don't have measurement instruments on hand, use visual cues to approximate portion proportions. As an example:

A dish of meat, poultry, or fish is roughly the size of a deck of cards or your palm.

A carbohydrate serving, such as rice or pasta, is roughly the size of a clenched hand.

A handful of nuts or seeds is one serving. Divide your dish into sections to manage portion sizes. Visualize splitting your plate into sections to control portion sizes.

Non-starchy veggies such as leafy greens, broccoli, or peppers should account for half of your meal.

A quarter of your dish should be devoted to a lean protein source such as chicken, fish, or tofu. The remaining quarter should be reserved for complex carbs such as whole grains or starchy vegetables.

Be wary of Calorie-dense Foods: Some foods contain more calories than others, even in tiny amounts. Keep oils, dressings, sauces, and sweets in mind. To minimize calorie consumption, use them sparingly or pick lighter alternatives.

Practice mindful eating: Mindful eating entails paying attention to your body's hunger and fullness cues. Eat gently, savoring each meal, and stopping when you're satisfied but not stuffed.

Be aware of eating out: When dining out, keep in mind that restaurants sometimes provide greater servings than necessary. To avoid overeating, consider sharing a meal with a friend or storing leftovers for later.

Remember that portion control is only one part of calorie management. It's also crucial to pay attention to the quality of your meal choices, choose nutrient-dense foods, and pay attention to your body's hunger and fullness cues. Maintaining a balanced and mindful eating style will help with general health and weight control.

Recommended supplements for endomorphs

Protein Powder for Muscle recovery and Growth

Protein powder can be a handy and efficient supplement for muscle repair and growth, particularly for people who struggle to fulfill their protein needs from whole food sources alone. Here are some important details concerning protein powder and its advantages:

Protein source: Protein powder supplements are commonly prepared from whey, casein, soy, pea, hemp, or rice protein sources. Each protein source has its own specific digestion rate, amino acid composition, and allergenic risk. Select a protein powder that is appropriate for your dietary habits, tolerances, and objectives.

Muscle recovery: Protein is essential for muscle repair and recovery following strenuous exercise. Consuming protein powder after an exercise can provide a quick amount of amino acids to kick-start the muscle repair process and maximize recovery.

Muscle growth: Protein is the building block of muscle tissue, so getting enough of it is critical for muscle growth. Protein powder can help you meet your protein objectives by supplementing your daily protein consumption, especially if you have increased protein requirements due to rigorous exercise or specialized fitness goals.

Convenience and Versatility: Protein powder is simple to use. It may be combined with water or another drink to make a fast and portable protein shake. Protein powder may also be added to a variety of dishes, such as smoothies, protein bars, or baked goods, to boost the protein value of your meals and snacks.

Timing And Dosage: It is typically suggested to drink protein powder within 30 minutes to an hour after your workout to help muscle healing and development. Aim for a portion size that contains 20–30 grams of protein per meal, while individual protein requirements may differ depending on factors such as body weight, activity level, and objectives.

Considerations: While protein powder can be advantageous, it should be used to enhance a well-balanced diet rather than to replace entire food sources of protein. Whole foods include extra nutrients, fiber, and other beneficial substances that are necessary for good health. Also, keep track of your overall protein intake from food and supplements, since too much protein can be harmful to your health.

Choosing a high-quality product: When shopping for protein powder, look for reputed brands that have been subjected to third-party testing for quality and purity. Check product labels for extra components such as sweeteners, flavors, or additives, and select alternatives that match your preferences and dietary requirements.

Keep in mind that protein powder is a supplement that should be taken in conjunction with a healthy diet and frequent exercise. Consult a healthcare practitioner, licensed dietitian, or sports nutritionist to assess your particular protein requirements and verify that protein powder supplementation is consistent with your overall health and fitness objectives.

Essential Vitamins and Minerals to support overall Health

It is critical to ensure a sufficient intake of key vitamins and minerals to promote overall health. Here are several important vitamins and minerals, as well as their significance in general health:

Vitamin A: Essential for vision, immune function, and cell growth and development. Good sources include carrots, sweet potatoes, spinach, and liver.

Vitamin C: Important for immune function, collagen synthesis, and antioxidant protection. Found in citrus fruits, berries, bell peppers, and leafy greens.

Vitamin D: Crucial for bone health, immune function, and calcium absorption. Sunlight exposure, fortified dairy products, fatty fish, and egg yolks are sources of vitamin D.

Vitamin E: Acts as an antioxidant, supporting cell protection and immune function. Nuts, seeds, vegetable oils, and leafy greens are sources of vitamin E.

Vitamin K: Essential for blood clotting and bone health. Found in leafy greens, broccoli, and fermented foods.

B-vitamins (B1, B2, B3, B5, B6, B7, B9, B12): Play roles in energy metabolism, nerve function, red blood cell production, and DNA synthesis. Sources include whole grains, legumes, nuts, seeds, lean meats, and dairy products.

Calcium: Vital for bone health, muscle function, and nerve transmission. Dairy products, leafy greens, tofu, and fortified plant-based milk are calcium sources.

Magnesium: Involved in hundreds of biochemical reactions, including energy production, muscle and nerve function, and bone health. Good sources include nuts, seeds, legumes, leafy greens, and whole grains.

Iron: Necessary for oxygen transport, energy production, and immune function. Red meat, poultry, fish, legumes, and leafy greens are iron-rich foods.

Zinc: Supports immune function, wound healing, and DNA synthesis. Shellfish, red meat, poultry, legumes, and nuts are sources of zinc.

Potassium: Important for heart health, fluid balance, and muscle function. Bananas, potatoes, citrus fruits, tomatoes, and leafy greens are potassium-rich foods.

Omega-3 Fatty Acids: Essential for brain health, heart health, and reducing inflammation. Fatty fish (such as salmon and sardines), flaxseeds, chia seeds, and walnuts are good sources.

It's worth mentioning that these are only a few of the numerous vitamins and minerals needed for good health. A varied and balanced diet rich in fruits, vegetables, whole grains, lean meats, and healthy fats is essential for acquiring these nutrients. Individual nutritional requirements may vary; therefore, it's always a good idea to get tailored advice and assistance from a healthcare expert or registered dietitian.

CHAPTER SEVEN

MOTIVATION AND SUPPORT FOR ENDOMORPHS

Overcoming Plateaus and staying consistent

Strategies for breaking through Training and Nutrition Plateaus

Breaking through training and dietary plateaus might be difficult, but you can do it with the appropriate tactics. Here are a few excellent ways to break through plateaus:

Change your training variables: Plateaus are common when your body adjusts to your existing training regimen. You may combat this by modifying your training factors such as intensity, volume, frequency, and exercise selection. In order to offer novel stimulation to your muscles, incorporate new exercises, raise weights, adjust rep ranges, or change the sequence of your workouts.

Attempt new training approaches: Trying new training techniques will help you push your body in new ways. Drop sets, supersets, pyramids, tempo training, and rest-pause sets are some examples. These approaches can spice up your exercises and promote muscular growth.

Increase your exercise intensity: Working harder throughout your sessions will help you break past plateaus. This can be accomplished by raising the weight, decreasing rest periods, including high-intensity interval training (HIIT), or incorporating advanced training techniques like forced reps or negatives.

Periodize your training: Periodization is the practice of varying training intensity, volume, and exercise selection over a specified period of time. This systematic method helps to avoid plateaus by constantly challenging your body while also allowing for proper recuperation. You may split your training into stages like hypertrophy, strength, and power, each with its own set of goals.

Modify your Nutrition: Make changes to your nutrition if you've reached a stalemate in your nutrition improvement. Consume a well-balanced diet rich in protein, healthy fats, and complex carbs. Adjust your calorie consumption in accordance with your goals, and consider tracking your food intake to verify you're staying within a healthy calorie range. In addition, evaluate your macronutrient ratios and make any necessary adjustments.

Change your eating pattern: If you've been following a certain eating pattern or meal time, such as intermittent fasting, you can experiment with changing it to see if it helps you break through the plateau. Changing the timing of your meals or adopting new eating patterns might sometimes help your success.

Seek expert help: If you've done everything and are still stuck at a plateau, go to a certified personal trainer or registered nutritionist. They can provide you with individualized advice and design a training and nutrition plan that is suited to your unique requirements and goals.

Maintain consistency and motivation: Plateaus might be mentally taxing, but it's critical to maintain consistency and motivation. Concentrate on your long-term goals, enjoy minor triumphs along the way, and remind yourself of your previous accomplishments. To help you stay accountable and motivated, surround yourself with a supportive network of friends, family, or like-minded people.

plateaus are a natural part of any fitness quest. You may break through plateaus and continue making progress toward your intended outcomes by applying these tactics and being dedicated to your goals.

Developing a resilient and dedicated mentality

Building a resilient and dedicated mentality is essential for long-term success in any fitness program. Here are some techniques for developing a resilient and committed mindset:

Set clear goals: Define your fitness objectives and break them down into smaller, more manageable milestones. Having specific goals gives you direction and drive, helping you stay focused and committed.

Develop a good attitude: Adopt a positive attitude and believe in your abilities to overcome obstacles. Adopt a growth attitude, in which you see challenges as chances for development and progress.

Accept the process: Recognize that improvement requires time and effort. Accept the trip and concentrate on the process rather than the ultimate result. Celebrate the tiny triumphs and acknowledge the everyday progress you make.

Maintain your Dedication: Dedication necessitates consistency and commitment. Make a program and stick to your training and diet regimens. Prioritize your health and well-being by making fitness a priority in your life.

Find your Motivation: Figure out what inspires you and use it as fuel to keep going. It might be a yearning for greater health, more vitality, more self-confidence, or just a desire to move. To stay on track, remind yourself of your motivation on a frequent basis.

Surround yourself with support: Create a network of like-minded people who can inspire and motivate you. Join fitness forums, find a workout partner, or seek advice from a coach or trainer. Surrounding oneself with good influences can assist you in being resilient and committed.

Learn from failures: Failures and challenges are unavoidable. Instead of being disheartened, look at them as chances to grow. Analyze what went wrong, make any necessary adjustments, and keep moving ahead. Setbacks can be used as stepping stones to future achievement.

Practice self-care: Maintain your general well-being by practicing self-care. Get enough sleep, control your stress, and emphasize rest and recuperation. Feed your body nourishing foods and engage in self-care activities that will revitalize your mind and body.

Track your progress: Keep a log of your progress to keep track of your accomplishments. Keep track of your exercises, measurements, and achievements. Visible proof of your success may improve your motivation and strengthen your commitment.

Stay inspired: Stay inspired Look for inspiration from individuals who have accomplished similar goals or overcome obstacles. Read success stories, follow fitness influencers, and watch inspiring videos. Use these sources of motivation to keep yourself motivated and to remind yourself that your objectives are reachable.

Remember that developing resilience and devotion is an ongoing process. Embrace the adventure, stay committed to your objectives, and develop a mentality that will help you overcome challenges and prosper on your fitness journey.

Monitoring progress and rewarding achievements

Using measuring instruments and taking progress pictures

Using measuring tools and progress images to track your fitness progress and provide visual evidence of your transformation may be beneficial. Here's how to use these tools effectively:

Body measurements: Using a tape measure, take frequent body measurements to document changes in certain regions of your body. Chest, waist, hips, thighs, and arms are common measures. Keep track of these metrics in a notebook or spreadsheet.

Body weight: Use a reputable scale to weigh yourself on a regular basis and record your weight in a diary or monitoring app. Remember that weight alone does not offer a comprehensive picture of your development because it does not distinguish between muscle and fat. It can, however, be beneficial to track overall patterns and changes over time.

Body fat percentage: To assess your body fat percentage, use body fat calipers or bioelectrical impedance instruments. This measurement gives you information about your body composition and can help you track changes in muscle and fat mass. It's crucial to remember that while these approaches may have some tolerance for error, when used regularly, they may be a valuable tool for measuring development.

Take frequent progress shots from several angles (front, back, and side) with constant lighting and attire. These photographs show the progression of your body's changes throughout time. Compare your photographs side by side to see how muscle definition, general shape, and body composition have changed.

Strength and performance measures: Track your strength and performance in the gym in addition to physical measurements. Keep track of how much weight you lift, how many repetitions you do, and how long it takes you to finish various exercises or programs. Tracking your strength increases and performance improvements may be extremely motivating and indicative of progress.

Maintain a fitness notebook in which you may record your exercises, nutrition, ideas, and feelings about your progress. Use this notebook to reflect on your journey, keep track of your achievements, and discover opportunities for growth. Reviewing your diary entries on a regular basis can reveal insights into your thinking, habits, and general growth.

Keep in mind that these measuring tools and progress images are only one component of tracking your progress. It's critical to examine how you feel, your energy levels, and your general fitness and well-being gains. The combination of quantitative data and subjective observations will provide you with a comprehensive picture of your fitness improvement.

Recognizing accomplishments and rewarding oneself for reaching milestones

Recognizing accomplishments and rewarding yourself for milestones is a vital part of staying motivated and enjoying your fitness success. Here are some ideas for rewarding yourself and recognizing your accomplishments:

Set Milestone Objectives: Break your major fitness goals down into smaller, more manageable benchmarks. These might be based on particular measures, performance goals, or following your training and diet plan. Celebrate each milestone as a great accomplishment along the way.

Non-Food Incentives: Instead of using food as a reward, choose non-food rewards that correspond to your interests and desires. Purchase new exercise attire, a massage, a spa day, a new fitness device, or a book you've been meaning to read. Choose incentives that will encourage and thrill you while also contributing to your general well-being.

Organize Special Activities: As you hit key milestones, organize pleasurable activities that will help you feel more accomplished and well-adjusted. It may be a weekend vacation, a trek in the woods, a new fitness class, or a day of pampering. These events might act as lasting reminders of the excellent lifestyle choices you've made.

Document and Reflect on Accomplishments: Take the time to document and recognize your accomplishments. Write them down in a notebook or make a visual depiction of your milestones and triumphs, such as a progress board or collage. Reflecting on how far you've come may improve your confidence and inspire you to keep going.

Share your triumphs with others: Share your achievements with encouraging friends, family, or an online fitness group. Their encouraging remarks and support can help reinforce your success while also providing a sense of reward and validation.

Self-care is important; therefore, prioritize self-care activities that promote relaxation and renewal. Schedule frequent self-care techniques, such as taking a bubble bath, practicing mindfulness or meditation, obtaining a good night's sleep, or participating in an enjoyable activity. Taking care of your physical and emotional health is a satisfying way to commemorate your trip.

Reflect on Personal Progress: Not only should you celebrate physical changes but also personal growth and beneficial habits that you've formed along the way. Recognize the discipline, devotion, and tenacity you've shown. Recognize the beneficial influence your fitness journey has had on other aspects of your life, such as greater confidence, higher energy, or improved stress management.

Remember that awards should be relevant and in line with your beliefs and objectives. They should serve to encourage your commitment to a healthy lifestyle as well as give positive reinforcement for your accomplishments. By rewarding yourself for accomplishments, you establish a positive feedback loop that drives motivation and promotes continuous growth on your fitness path.

Finding responsibility and support in Fitness Communities

Joining fitness organizations, participating in internet forums, or hiring a personal trainer

Endomorphs might greatly benefit from joining fitness organizations, internet forums, or engaging a personal trainer on their fitness quest. Here are some examples of how each choice may provide guidance, incentive, and support:

Fitness groups: Joining local fitness organizations or clubs helps you connect with other people who have similar goals and struggles. These organizations frequently provide group workouts, training sessions, and social gatherings where you may meet new people, make exercise buddies, and share ideas and advice. A supportive group may offer accountability, encouragement, and a sense of belonging, making your fitness journey more fun and sustainable.

Online forums: Participating in online fitness forums and communities allows you to connect with people from all over the world who share your fitness interests and experiences. These discussion boards are excellent for getting help, sharing progress, addressing problems, and learning from others. You may get new insights, gain access to a plethora of knowledge, and receive support from a broad group of people who have experienced similar challenges and discovered successful solutions.

Personal trainer: Hiring a personal trainer may provide you with individualized assistance, knowledge, and accountability that are geared to your unique requirements and goals. A certified personal trainer can analyze your body type, create a personalized training plan, teach appropriate form and technique, measure your progress, and give continuous encouragement and support. They may also assist you in breaking through plateaus, adjusting your workout program as needed, and providing dietary advice to supplement your training efforts.

Joining a fitness organization, participating in online forums, or hiring a personal trainer are all choices that may provide useful information and support. They offer the opportunity to learn from others, obtain fresh ideas, seek expert advice, and stay encouraged on your fitness quest. Remember to choose an option that corresponds to your interests, budget, and accessibility, and to be open to the connections and information that these communities may bring.

Participating in social support for motivation and encouragement

Endomorphs can get encouragement, inspiration, and accountability on their fitness path by engaging in social support. Here are some strategies for actively seeking and leveraging social support:

Find a workout buddy: Working out with a friend, family member, or coworker who has similar fitness objectives to you will help you stay motivated and enjoy your exercises. You may plan and engage in exercises together, as well as support and hold each other responsible.

Join online fitness communities: There are several fitness communities available on online platforms and social media where you can connect with people who share your interests and ambitions. Join groups, follow fitness influencers, and participate in discussions to get advice, share your progress, and find inspiration. Even from a distance, these networks may provide a sense of kinship and support.

Attend exercise courses or group workouts: Attending fitness classes or group workouts at your local gym, studio, or community center helps you connect with other fitness enthusiasts. These group settings offer a helpful and inspiring environment in which you may engage with others, exchange experiences, and encourage one another to do your best.

Share your journey on social media: Create a fitness-focused social media account to share your progress, exercises, and observations. Engage with others in the fitness community by commenting on their postings, offering encouragement, and congratulating them on their accomplishments. Throughout your fitness journey, this virtual network may provide a sense of camaraderie and encouragement.

Seek help from friends and family: Tell your friends and family about your fitness objectives and success. Let them know how they can help you, whether it's with encouraging words, accompanying you in exercises, or keeping you accountable. Their understanding and support might be important in keeping you motivated and focused.

Consider a fitness coach or mentor: Working with a fitness coach or mentor who specializes in endomorph training can provide professional direction and tailored assistance. They may assist you with navigating obstacles, setting realistic objectives, and providing continual encouragement and responsibility.

Know that social assistance is a two-way street. Be willing to help others in their fitness pursuits. You can build a pleasant and uplifting environment that feeds everyone's achievement by cultivating a community of support and motivation.

CHAPTER EIGHT

RECOVERY AND INJURY PREVENTION

Importance of rest and recovery days

Understanding the role of rest in muscle repair and growth

Rest is an essential component of muscle repair and development for endomorphs and people of all body types. Here's a quick rundown of the importance of rest in muscle recovery:

Muscle repair: Muscles sustain microscopic injury and disintegration during exercise, particularly strength training. Rest intervals help the body begin the healing process. Damaged muscle fibers are healed and regenerated during this time, resulting in muscular development and greater strength. The body is unable to repair and rebuild muscles adequately without proper rest, which might stymie growth.

Hormonal balance: Rest is crucial for maintaining hormonal equilibrium, which includes the release of growth hormone and testosterone, both of which are required for muscular growth and development. Adequate rest enables proper hormone synthesis, allowing the body to efficiently develop and repair muscle tissue.

Energy restoration: Intense workouts deplete the body's energy resources, such as glycogen, which serves as the major source of fuel for muscles. Rest helps the body restore its energy stores, ensuring that it has the resources it needs to promote muscle repair and growth throughout the following activities.

Injury avoidance: Rest intervals allow the body to recuperate from the stress and strain of exercise, lowering the chance of overuse problems. Continuous and hard training without enough rest can result in tiredness, lower performance, and an increased risk of injury, all of which can stymie development.

Rest days should be included in your training plan to improve muscle regeneration and development. This encompasses both active rest, which comprises low-intensity activities like walking or stretching, and full rest, which involves no planned activity. Individual factors such as training intensity, recovery ability, and general fitness level may influence the frequency and duration of rest days. It is advised that you take at least one to two days off every week to allow your muscles and body to recuperate and adjust to the training stimulus.

Remember that rest is not a sign of weakness or a lack of commitment; it is an important aspect of the entire training process. By putting rest and recovery first, you give your muscles the time and resources they need to heal and grow, resulting in better performance and success on your fitness path.

Methods for combining active recovery and relaxation approaches

As an endomorph, incorporating active recovery and relaxation strategies into your regimen can improve muscle recovery and general well-being. Consider the following strategies:

Low-impact activities: On rest days or as part of your active recovery plan, engage in low-impact activities. Walking, swimming, yoga, Pilates, and mild cycling are examples of such hobbies. These activities increase blood circulation, aid in the removal of metabolic waste from the muscles, and provide a moderate kind of movement to aid in recuperation.

Stretching and mobility exercises: Stretching and mobility activities, such as dynamic stretching, static stretching, and foam rolling, should be prioritized. These exercises can help with flexibility, range of motion, and muscular tension. Stretch the key muscle groups that you worked on throughout your strength training workouts.

Mind-body practices: Incorporate mind-body activities into your routine, such as meditation, deep breathing exercises, or mindfulness. These routines can aid in stress reduction, relaxation, and mental clarity. Consider devoting a few minutes each day to these habits in order to improve your general well-being.

Active recovery workouts: Instead of full idleness on your rest days, consider doing light workouts that target different muscle groups or focus on different types of exercise. Try a mild yoga session, a short swim, or a leisurely bike ride, for example. These exercises increase blood flow and give your body a respite from hard strength training while still allowing it to heal.

Massage or self-myofascial release: To target tight muscles and relieve tension, receive a massage or utilize self-myofascial release techniques like foam rolling or massage balls. These techniques can boost circulation, relieve muscular pain, and induce relaxation.

Adequate sleep: Make obtaining adequate quality sleep each night a priority. Sleep is essential for muscle healing as well as general wellness. To allow your body to recover and renew, aim for 7-9 hours of uninterrupted sleep every night.

Remember to listen to your body and discover the right balance of active recovery and relaxation strategies for you. Incorporating these tactics into your regimen will not only aid in muscle repair and growth but will also benefit your entire well-being as an endomorph.

Mobility and stretching exercises

Incorporating dynamic and static stretching routines

Endomorphs can greatly benefit from including both dynamic and static stretching workouts into their training program. Here's a summary of each form of stretching and how to successfully utilize it:

Dynamic stretching: Dynamic stretching entails vigorous motions that take muscles and joints through their entire range of motion. It improves flexibility and prepares the body for physical exertion by increasing blood flow. Stretch dynamically before your exercise or strength-training session. Here are some dynamic stretching examples:

Leg swings: Stand next to a support and swing one leg forward and backward, increasing the range of motion progressively. Rep on the other side

Extend your arms out to the sides and create forward and backward circles, gradually increasing the size of the circles.

Walking lunges: Take a step forward into a lunge, keeping your front knee exactly above your ankle. As you move ahead, alternate your legs. Each dynamic stretch should be done 10–15 times, or for a distance of 10–15 meters.

Arm circles: Extend your arms out to the sides and make circles in a forward and backward motion, gradually increasing the size of the circles.

Static stretching: Static stretching is keeping a stretch position for a lengthy amount of time, often 20–30 seconds, without any bouncing or movement. Static stretching improves flexibility, lengthens muscles, and promotes calm. Static stretching should be done at the end of your workout or strength training session. Here are some static stretch examples:

Hamstring stretch: Stretch your hamstrings by sitting on the floor with one leg stretched in front of you and the other bent. Lean forward from your hips and grasp your toes.

Chest stretch: To feel a stretch in your chest and shoulders, stand near a doorway, lay your forearm on the doorframe, and slowly move your body away from the arm.

Quadriceps stretch: Stretch your quadriceps by standing up and grabbing one ankle with one hand, dragging your heel towards your glutes until you feel a stretch in the front of your thigh. Hold each static stretch for 20–30 seconds to provide a moderate, regulated stretch that is free of pain or discomfort.

Remember to warm up your muscles and prepare them for activity by performing dynamic stretches before your workout. To help calm down the body and enhance flexibility, save static stretching until the end of your workout. Listen to your body, avoid pushing yourself into discomfort, and adjust stretches as needed based on your specific flexibility and comfort level.

Increasing flexibility and avoiding muscle imbalances

Endomorphs must improve their flexibility and avoid muscular imbalances in order to improve their general fitness and lower their chance of injury. Here are some ideas to add to your daily routine:

Stretching exercises: Regular stretching improves flexibility and helps your joints maintain a balanced range of motion. Stretch the hamstrings, quadriceps, hip flexors, calves, chest, shoulders, and back, among other key muscle groups. Hold each stretch for 20–30 seconds and repeat at least two to three times each week.

Mobility exercises: Include mobility exercises that target specific joints and muscle groups to improve their range of motion. Hip circles, shoulder dislocations, ankle rotations, and spinal twists are a few examples. Regularly perform these exercises to preserve joint mobility and avoid muscle stiffness.

Corrective exercises: identify and integrate corrective workouts to treat any muscular imbalances or areas of weakness. If you have weak glutes, for example, consider glute bridges and hip thrusts to strengthen them. Exercises such as lunges and hip flexor stretches can help lengthen and release tight hip flexors.

Balance training: Exercises that stress your balance and proprioception should be included in your balance training. This aids in the improvement of stability, coordination, and neuromuscular control. Single-leg squats, standing on one leg, and utilizing a balancing board can all help.

Yoga or Pilates: Consider including yoga or Pilates into your workout program. These exercises emphasize strength, flexibility, and body awareness, which aid in general mobility and the prevention of imbalances.

Self-myofascial release and foam rolling: Use a foam roller or other self-massage equipment to relieve tension and knots in muscles and fascia. This can assist in enhancing flexibility, decreasing muscular tension, and correcting any imbalances.

Postural awareness: Postural awareness means paying attention to your posture throughout the day, both during workouts and during daily tasks. To promote excellent posture, practice maintaining optimal alignment and using your core muscles.

You may enhance flexibility, resolve muscle imbalances, and promote general musculoskeletal health by implementing these tactics into your training program. Remember to begin cautiously, listen to your body, and seek the advice of a trained fitness expert if necessary.

Managing and Preventing Common Strength Training Injuries

Proper warm-up and cool-down routines

Endomorphs require proper warm-up and cool-down routines to prepare their bodies for activity and facilitate recovery afterward. Here are some pointers to keep in mind:

1. Warm-up:

General cardiovascular warm-up: Warm up your cardiovascular system by doing 5–10 minutes of modest aerobic activity such as brisk walking, running, or cycling. This raises your heart rate and body temperature, preparing you for more strenuous action.

Dynamic stretching: Perform dynamic stretches that entail controlled motions over the whole range of motion. This promotes increased blood flow, muscular activation, and joint mobility. Leg swings, arm circles, walking lunges, and hip rotations are a few examples.

Activation exercises: These exercises target particular muscle areas that will be used during your workout. These workouts aid in muscular activation, brain activation, and stability. Include movements like bodyweight squats or glute bridges in a leg workout, for example, to stimulate lower body muscles.

Sport-specific warm-up: If you're participating in a specific sport or activity, integrate movements that mirror the demands of that activity. If you play basketball, for example, add some dribbling, shooting, and lateral movements to your warm-up.

2. Relaxation:

Gradual cooldown: Once you've finished your workout, gently reduce the intensity of your activities. This helps your heart rate and body temperature gradually return to normal.

Static stretching: Include static stretches in which you hold each stretch for around 20–30 seconds. Stretch the muscles that were worked on throughout your workout. This aids in the improvement of flexibility and the prevention of muscular stiffness.

Foam rolling: Roll over the major muscle groups using a foam roller or other self-massage equipment. This can aid in the release of tension, the improvement of blood circulation, and the reduction of post-workout muscular soreness.

Deep breathing and relaxation: Set aside some time to practice deep breathing and relaxation techniques. This can help relax and heal the nervous system by calming it down.

Warm-up and cool-down exercises help your body prepare for activity, lower the chance of injury, increase performance, and aid in post-workout recovery. Remember to customize your warm-up and cool-down exercises to the sort of activity or workout you'll be performing.

Listening to the body and seeking expert assistance if necessary

Endomorphs must pay attention to their bodies on their fitness quest. During activity, be alert to any indicators of exhaustion, discomfort, or pain. If you are experiencing prolonged pain or discomfort, you should seek the advice of a healthcare expert or a competent trainer to assess the situation and identify the best course of action.

Furthermore, if you're new to strength training or have special fitness objectives, consulting with a personal trainer or strength coach might be advantageous. They may offer specialized advice, design a customized training plan, guarantee perfect form and technique, and assist you in progressing safely and successfully.

A competent practitioner can also help you adapt workouts or routines to meet physical limits or prevent injuries. They can offer essential advice on the correct diet, supplements, and lifestyle changes to help you achieve your objectives.

Remember that every person's fitness path is different, and it's critical to prioritize your health and well-being. If you have any worries or questions, don't be afraid to seek the advice and assistance of specialists who can help you along the way.

CONCLUSION

RECAP OF KEY POINTS AND TAKEAWAYS

Understanding the endomorph body type and its challenges

To properly meet the requirements of people with this body type, it is essential to understand the endomorph body type and its problems. Here are some important things to think about:

Definition of Endomorph Body Type:

Endomorphs are characterized by a naturally higher body fat percentage, a slower metabolism, and a tendency to store fat easily. They typically look rounder and softer, have wider bones, and are more likely to gain weight quickly.

Challenges Faced by Endomorphs:

Endomorphs often face challenges when it comes to losing weight and gaining muscle. Their slower metabolic rate makes it more difficult to burn calories and shed excess body fat. They could also be more prone to hormonal imbalances and insulin resistance, which can make managing their weight more difficult.

Weight Loss Plateaus: Because endomorphs' bodies are more likely to adapt to dietary and exercise changes, they may experience weight loss plateaus more frequently. Although this may be discouraging, it's crucial to be persistent and patient.

Fat storage places: Endomorphs usually have distinct places where fat prefers to build, such as the belly, hips, and thighs. Targeting these areas with exercise and nutrition strategies can help address these concerns.

Importance of Strength Training, Proper Nutrition, and Recovery

Strength training, proper nutrition, and recovery are all vital components for achieving optimal health, fitness, and body composition. Here's why each of these elements is crucial:

Strength Training: Strength training plays a crucial role in creating lean muscle mass, enhancing strength, and boosting metabolism. Strength training can be especially helpful for endomorphs, who may have a slower metabolic rate and a propensity to store body fat. By engaging in resistance exercises like weightlifting, you can stimulate muscle growth, which in turn increases your resting metabolic rate and helps you burn more calories even at rest. Additionally, strength training improves bone density, changes movement patterns to be more functional, and improves overall body composition.

Proper nutrition: Nutrition is the cornerstone of every successful fitness regimen. It's crucial for endomorphs to concentrate on eating a balanced diet that promotes muscle building and fat reduction. Give nutrient-rich foods like lean proteins, whole grains, fruits, veggies, and healthy fats top priority. For muscle growth and repair, adequate protein consumption is especially important. Managing body weight and composition requires balancing macronutrients, managing portion sizes, and limiting calorie intake. Keep in mind to drink enough water and think about including the right supplements to support your nutritional needs.

Recovery: Recovery is often overlooked but essential for progress and injury prevention. When you engage in strength training, your muscles undergo stress and micro-tears, and proper recovery allows them to repair and grow stronger. To allow for appropriate recuperation, make sure to include rest days in your training regimen. Additionally, emphasize sleep, since it is vital for hormone control, muscle regeneration, and general well-being. Stretching, foam rolling, and massage are relaxation techniques that can help reduce muscle soreness and speed up recovery. You can train at your best and lower your risk of overuse injuries by taking good care of your body through rest and recovery.

Strength training, healthy eating, and enough rest and recovery all work together to produce a comprehensive fitness program that maximizes muscle growth, aids in fat reduction, and enhances general health. Remember to consult with professionals, such as trainers and nutritionists, to tailor your approach to your specific needs and goals.

Encouragement for Endomorphs on their fitness travels

Focusing on improvement over perfection

When beginning a fitness journey as an endomorph, it's crucial to prioritize progress over perfection. Here's why adopting this mindset is crucial:

Sustainable Approach: Pursuing perfection may result in exaggerated standards and an "all-or-nothing" outlook. This kind of thinking frequently leads to frustration, exhaustion, and a higher risk of giving up on your fitness objectives. Instead, concentrate on improving over time. Celebrate small victories, whether it's increasing the weight you lift, improving your endurance, or making healthier food choices. By acknowledging and appreciating your progress, you build momentum and maintain a long-term commitment to your fitness journey.

Consistency and Habit Formation: Progress is achieved through persistent effort and the development of good habits. Prioritize developing dependable routines that fit your lifestyle rather than striving for perfection. Consistent engagement in strength training, following a balanced nutrition plan, and practicing self-care strategies will yield greater results in the long run. It's the accumulation of tiny, persistent activities that leads to substantial modifications over time.

Motivation and Enjoyment: Focusing on progress encourages you to stay motivated and enjoy the process. There will be periods when progress seems slow or stagnant on fitness journeys. You may have a good outlook and find inspiration to keep moving forward by recognizing the progress you've already accomplished. Your fitness journey can also be more sustained and fulfilling if you find enjoyment in the activities you partake in, whether it's trying out new exercises, learning about various workout styles, or experimenting with healthy recipes.

Adaptability and Learning: Placing an emphasis on progress rather than perfection fosters flexibility and a readiness to draw lessons from failure. Recognize that setbacks are a natural part of any journey, and use them as opportunities for growth and learning. Adapt your strategy, get assistance when necessary, and keep trying out various tactics until you discover the one that works best for you. You can overcome obstacles, make necessary corrections, and keep moving toward your goals by adopting a growth mindset.

Keep in mind that every person's road to fitness is distinct, and progress looks different for everyone. By emphasizing progress over perfection, you create a positive and sustainable mindset that supports your growth, keeps you motivated, and helps you achieve long-term success as an endomorph.

Motivation to embrace the process and achieve long-term results

In order to embrace the process and produce lasting results as an endomorph, motivation is a crucial component. Following are some tips for maintaining motivation during your fitness journey:

Create Meaningful Goals: Create goals that have meaning for you personally. Make sure your goals are in line with your aspirations and moral principles, whether they include reducing a specific percentage of body fat, increasing muscle mass, increasing strength, or boosting general fitness. Your motivation and determination to stick with your goals can be increased by having a compelling "why" for doing them.

Break It Down: This makes it easier for you to monitor your progress and gives you a feeling of accomplishment as you go. Celebrate each accomplishment, no matter how minor, since it will keep you motivated and give you more self-assurance.

Find Your Why: Decide why you want to change and reach your fitness objectives. Maybe it's to raise your self-confidence, your energy levels, your health, or your general quality of life. It's simpler to stay motivated and overcome obstacles when you have a clear understanding of why you're on this journey.

Make Your Environment Supportive: Surround yourself with people who share your goals and who will encourage you. Join online forums, make contact with exercise partners, or look for local groups where you can discuss your successes and setbacks. Your motivation and accountability can significantly change if you have a support system.

Track Your Progress: Keep a log of your workouts, diet, and measurements to track your progress. Being able to see the concrete results of your efforts can be highly motivating. Take pictures, assess your body's composition, keep tabs on your strength gains, and make note of any improvements to your general wellbeing. These visual cues act as a strong motivator and aid in maintaining your attention on the long-term outcomes.

Mix It Up: Add variety to your routine to break up the monotony and keep your workouts interesting. Try new gym courses, experiment with different routines, or engage in outdoor pursuits. You can avoid boredom and maintain interest in your exercise journey by adding variation.

Celebrate Non-Scale Victories: Don't just look at the weight on the scale to determine your success. Recognize and celebrate non-scale victories such as increased energy, improved sleep, enhanced mood, or achieving new personal bests in your workouts. These triumphs give you more drive to keep going on your path since they show that you've made progress beyond just changing your weight or measurements.

Practice self-care: Take care of your total well-being by emphasizing self-care. Get enough rest, control your stress, and pay attention to your body's needs. Taking time to rest and recover properly will prevent burnout and keep your motivation levels high.

Remember, motivation is not always constant, and it's normal to experience fluctuations in your drive. When you're lacking motivation, review your objectives, reaffirm your motivation, and look for role models or success stories in the fitness industry for motivation. You can embrace the process and accomplish your fitness goals as an endomorph with a combination of self-motivation, a supportive environment, and a focus on long-term results.

Answers to Frequently Asked Questions

A. Can endomorphs grow lean muscular mass?

Endomorphs can absolutely increase their lean muscle mass. Despite having a stronger propensity to accumulate body fat, endomorphs may efficiently grow muscle and develop their ideal physiques with the appropriate approach to exercise and diet.

B. How often should endomorphs strength train?

The frequency of strength exercise for endomorphs depends on several aspects, including individual goals, recuperation capability, and training experience. As a general rule, aiming for at least 3–4 strength training sessions per week is a good place to start. However, it's important to listen to your body and allow for adequate rest and recovery between sessions.

C. What are the best dietary strategies for endomorphs?

For endomorphs, a balanced diet that emphasizes whole, nutrient-dense foods is key. Focus on consuming lean proteins, complex carbohydrates, and healthy fats in appropriate portions. Pay attention to your calorie intake, and if you want to lose fat, make a small calorie deficit. It's also essential to monitor macronutrient ratios and adjust them according to individual needs and preferences.

D. Can endomorphs incorporate cardio alongside strength training?

Absolutely. Incorporating cardiovascular exercises alongside strength training can be beneficial for endomorphs. Cardio can enhance calorie burn, improve cardiovascular health, and assist in fat reduction. Aim for a combination of moderate-intensity steady-state cardio and high-intensity interval training (HIIT) to maximize results.

E. How long does it take for an endomorph to see results from strength training?

As an endomorph, the time it takes to see results from strength training can vary depending on factors like personal genetics, training consistency, nutrition, and program adherence. With regular exercise and good nutrition, noticeable improvements in strength, muscle definition, and body composition can typically be seen within a few weeks to a few months. Please note that these are general answers to frequently asked questions, and individual experiences may vary. For personalized guidance based on your unique needs and circumstances, it is always advised to speak with a licensed fitness expert or healthcare provider.

F. Should endomorphs prioritize strength or cardio exercises?

Both cardio and strength training have their benefits for endomorphs. Lean muscle mass, which can boost metabolism and facilitate fat reduction, is developed through strength training. Cardiovascular exercises help burn calories and improve cardiovascular health. The optimal approach is to incorporate a combination of both cardio and strength training into your fitness routine to achieve balanced results and overall health.

G. How do endomorphs break through weight loss stalemates?

Anyone can experience a weight reduction plateau, including endomorphs. Consider using the following tactics to move past plateaus: **Adjust your caloric intake:** Evaluate your calorie intake and make sure you're still in a calorie deficit for weight loss. To meet your current metabolic demands, you might need to modify your calorie intake.

Change your workout program by adding new exercises, upping the intensity, or experimenting with new training techniques to push your body. Track your success. Monitor your progress closely by monitoring measurements, body composition, and strength increases. By doing this, you can spot potential plateaus and make the necessary corrections.

The key is to maintain consistency. Even if improvement seems to be taking a while, stick to your diet and exercise schedule. Continue forward and have faith in the process.

Seek support: Consider seeking guidance from a qualified fitness professional or joining a support group to gain motivation, accountability, and new perspectives on overcoming plateaus.

H. Supplements: Can they aid endomorphs in achieving their fitness goals?

Supplements can enhance an endomorph's well-rounded fitness program, though they are not a magic fix. Protein powders for muscle repair and development, omega-3 fatty acids for general health, and multivitamins to make up for any dietary deficiencies are a few supplements that may be helpful. However, it's important to note that supplements should not replace a balanced diet and proper nutrition. Always consult a healthcare expert before introducing any new supplements into your routine.

I. How can endomorphs maintain their motivation for exercising?

It might be difficult to stay motivated when trying to get in shape, but there are methods endomorphs can use to do so:

Establish clear, attainable objectives that are in line with your individual wants and aspirations. Break them down into smaller milestones to measure your progress and recognize victories along the way.

Identify accountability partners. Surround yourself with people who are encouraging and have similar fitness aspirations. This can be friends, family members, or joining fitness communities or online groups where you can connect with like-minded people.

Mix up your routine. Avoid monotony by incorporating variety into your workouts. To keep things fresh and challenging, try out new workouts, techniques, or classes.

Treat yourself as a reward for reaching milestones or maintaining a fitness regimen. Rewards may not have to involve food, such as purchasing new exercise equipment or treating yourself to a spa day.

Focus on the positive aspects of your journey, practice self-compassion, and give priority to self-care activities that help you unwind and reduce stress.

J. How can endomorphs sustainably control their body composition?

Long-term body composition management necessitates a sustainable strategy. Instead of relying on quick fixes, focus your attention on establishing healthy lifestyle habits. This includes consistent cardiovascular exercise for overall health, balanced nutrition that supports your goals, regular strength training to increase and maintain muscle mass, and a focus on rest and recovery. To maintain a healthy body composition over time, adopt a growth mindset and make adjustments as necessary. Keep in mind that these FAQs offer basic advice and information. It's important to consult with a qualified fitness professional or healthcare provider to address any specific concerns or individual needs.

Special Offer: As a valued reader, you will also receive bonus resources, including sample workout plans, exercise demonstrations, meal ideas, and a progress tracker, all designed to support your transformation and keep you on track.

BONUSES:

1. SAMPLE WORK OUT PLANS:

Sample Workout Plans for Endomorphs

Full-Body Strength Training Plan:

Workout Frequency: 3 times per week

Exercises: Squats, deadlifts, bench press, overhead press, pull-ups, lunges, planks

Sets and Reps: 3 sets of 8-12 reps for each exercise

Rest: 1-2 minutes between sets

Split Routine for Muscle Development:

Workout Frequency: 4-5 times per week

Day 1 (Upper Body): Bench press, rows, shoulder press, bicep curls, tricep dips

Day 2 (Lower Body): Squats, lunges, leg press, hamstring curls, calf raises

Day 3 (Rest)

Day 4 (Upper Body): Pull-ups, overhead press, lateral raises, tricep pushdowns, plank

Day 5 (Lower Body): Deadlifts, step-ups, glute bridges, leg extensions, Russian twists

Sets and Reps: 3-4 sets of 8-12 reps for each exercise

Rest: 1-2 minutes between sets

HIIT and Cardiovascular Training Plan:

Workout Frequency: 2-3 times per week

HIIT Workout: 20 minutes of high-intensity intervals (e.g., sprinting, burpees, mountain climbers) followed by 10 minutes of active recovery (e.g., walking, light jogging)

Cardiovascular Training: 30-45 minutes of moderate-intensity cardio (e.g., cycling, swimming, brisk walking) on alternate days

Rest: 1-2 days of complete rest per week

Functional Training Circuit:

Workout Frequency: 3-4 times per week

Circuit Exercises: Squat jumps, push-ups, kettlebell swings, box jumps, medicine ball slams, TRX rows

Perform each exercise for 30 seconds with minimal rest in between

Complete 3-4 rounds of the circuit

Rest: 1-2 minutes between circuits

Note: It is important to adjust the intensity, volume, and exercises based on your individual fitness level and any specific limitations or preferences you may have. Consult with a qualified fitness professional before starting any new workout program to ensure it aligns with your goals and capabilities.

2. EXERCISE DEMONSTRATION:

Here's a written illustration of an exercise demonstration:

1.Exercise: Squat

Step 1: Stand with your feet shoulder-width apart, toes pointing slightly outward. Engage your core and keep your chest lifted throughout the exercise.

Step 2: Begin the movement by bending your knees and pushing your hips back, as if you're sitting back into a chair. Keep your weight balanced on your heels.

Step 3: Lower your body down until your thighs are parallel to the ground or as low as your flexibility allows. Ensure your knees are in line with your toes and not extending beyond them.

Step 4: Pause briefly at the bottom position, then push through your heels to return to the starting position. Exhale as you rise.

Step 5: Repeat the movement for the desired number of repetitions.

Tips:

Keep your back straight and avoid rounding your shoulders.

Maintain a neutral spine throughout the exercise.

Engage your glutes and quadriceps as you push through your heels to stand back up.

Control the movement and avoid using momentum.

Variations:

Goblet Squat: Hold a dumbbell or kettlebell close to your chest with both hands, performing the squat in the same manner.

Sumo Squat: Widen your stance and point your toes out at a greater angle, emphasizing inner thigh engagement.

Bulgarian Split Squat: Elevate one foot behind you on a bench or step, lowering your body into a lunge position with the front leg.

Remember to consult with a fitness professional or trainer if you're new to exercise or have any concerns about performing the movements safely and effectively.

2. Exercise: Push-Up

Step 1: Start by positioning yourself face down on the floor with your hands slightly wider than shoulder-width apart. Place your toes on the ground, keeping your body in a straight line from head to toe. This is the starting position.

Step 2: Engage your core, squeeze your glutes, and lower your body towards the floor by bending your elbows. Keep your elbows tucked close to your body as you descend.

Step 3: Continue lowering your body until your chest is just above the ground or as low as your strength allows. Ensure your body remains straight without sagging or lifting your hips.

Step 4: Push through your palms and extend your arms to raise your body back to the starting position. Keep your core engaged throughout the movement.

Step 5: Repeat the movement for the desired number of repetitions.

Tips:

Maintain a neutral spine and avoid overarching or rounding your lower back.

Look slightly ahead to maintain proper alignment.

If the full push-up is challenging, modify by performing the exercise on your knees instead of your toes.

Keep a controlled pace and focus on engaging your chest, shoulders, and triceps muscles.

Variations:

Incline Push-Up: Place your hands on an elevated surface, such as a bench or step, to reduce the intensity of the exercise.

Decline Push-Up: Elevate your feet on a sturdy surface, such as a step or bench, to increase the challenge and engage your upper chest.

Wide Grip Push-Up: Position your hands wider than shoulder-width apart to emphasize your chest muscles.

Remember to listen to your body, start with an appropriate level of difficulty, and progress gradually as you build strength and confidence in the exercise. If you have any concerns or limitations, consult with a fitness professional for guidance.

3. Exercise: Dumbbell Squat

Step 1: Begin by standing with your feet shoulder-width apart, holding a dumbbell in each hand, arms hanging by your sides. This is your starting position.

Step 2: Engage your core, keep your chest lifted, and initiate the movement by bending your knees and lowering your hips back and down as if you're sitting into a chair. Imagine driving your heels into the ground to maintain stability.

Step 3: Continue descending until your thighs are parallel to the ground or as low as your mobility allows. Keep your knees tracking in line with your toes and your torso upright throughout the movement.

Step 4: Pause for a moment at the bottom position and then push through your heels to extend your knees and hips, returning to the starting position.

Step 5: Repeat the movement for the desired number of repetitions.

Tips:

Keep your chest lifted and your spine in a neutral position throughout the exercise.

Avoid letting your knees collapse inward or extend beyond your toes.

Maintain a slow and controlled movement, focusing on engaging your quadriceps, hamstrings, and glutes.

If holding dumbbells is challenging, you can perform the exercise without weights or use lighter dumbbells until you build strength.

Variations:

Goblet Squat: Hold a dumbbell vertically against your chest with both hands, allowing your elbows to point down. Perform the squat movement while maintaining a solid grip on the dumbbell.

Sumo Squat: Stand with your feet wider than shoulder-width apart and your toes turned out at an angle. Perform the squat by lowering your hips straight down, emphasizing your inner thighs and glutes.

Remember to always use proper form and start with a weight that challenges you without compromising your technique. As you become more comfortable with the exercise, you can gradually increase the weight or try different variations to target specific muscle groups. If you have any concerns or limitations, consult with a fitness professional for personalized guidance.

4. Exercise: Bench Press

Step 1: Lie flat on a bench with your feet firmly planted on the ground, shoulder-width apart. Grasp the barbell with an overhand grip slightly wider than shoulder-width apart. Lift the barbell off the rack and position it directly above your chest with your arms extended. This is your starting position.

Step 2: Lower the barbell slowly and under control towards your chest, keeping your elbows at a 45-degree angle to your body. Aim to touch the barbell to your chest lightly.

Step 3: Pause for a moment when the barbell reaches your chest, then press it back up to the starting position by extending your arms fully, while maintaining control and stability.

Step 4: Repeat the movement for the desired number of repetitions.

Tips:

Keep your back flat against the bench and your shoulder blades squeezed together throughout the exercise.

Ensure that your wrists are in a neutral position, aligned with your forearms.

Engage your core muscles to maintain stability and prevent excessive arching or lifting of the lower back.

Exhale as you press the barbell up and inhale as you lower it down.

Start with a weight that allows you to maintain proper form and gradually increase the weight as you become stronger.

Variations:

Dumbbell Bench Press: Instead of using a barbell, use dumbbells held in each hand. This allows for a greater range of motion and can help address any strength imbalances between your arms.

Incline Bench Press: Adjust the bench to a slight incline (around 30-45 degrees) to target the upper chest muscles more specifically.

Close-Grip Bench Press: Place your hands closer together on the barbell, with your thumbs almost touching. This variation emphasizes the triceps muscles.

Remember to always warm up properly before performing any exercise and consult with a fitness professional if you have any concerns or limitations. Proper form and technique are crucial for maximizing the benefits of the exercise while minimizing the risk of injury.

5. Exercise: Dumbbell Shoulder Press

Step 1: Start by sitting on a bench or an upright position with your back straight and your feet flat on the floor. Hold a dumbbell in each hand at shoulder level, palms facing forward. This is your starting position.

Step 2: Press the dumbbells overhead by extending your arms upward, while maintaining control and stability. Avoid locking out your elbows at the top of the movement.

Step 3: Pause briefly at the top, feeling the contraction in your shoulders and upper arms.

Step 4: Lower the dumbbells back to the starting position by bending your elbows and allowing the weights to come down to shoulder level.

Step 5: Repeat the movement for the desired number of repetitions.

Tips:

Keep your core engaged and maintain a neutral spine throughout the exercise.

Avoid excessive arching of the lower back or leaning back during the press.

Exhale as you press the dumbbells overhead and inhale as you lower them back down.

Start with lighter weights to establish proper form and gradually increase the weight as you become stronger.

Maintain control throughout the movement and avoid using momentum to lift the dumbbells.

Variations:

Seated Dumbbell Shoulder Press: Perform the exercise while seated on a bench or an adjustable seat with back support. This helps isolate the shoulder muscles and minimizes involvement from other muscle groups.

Arnold Press: Start the movement with your palms facing your body, then rotate the dumbbells as you press them overhead, so that your palms face forward at the top of the movement. This variation targets different areas of the shoulder muscles.

Single-Arm Dumbbell Shoulder Press: Perform the exercise one arm at a time, alternating between the left and right sides. This helps address any strength imbalances and requires greater stability.

Remember to use proper form, choose appropriate weights, and listen to your body. If you experience any pain or discomfort during the exercise, stop immediately and seek guidance from a qualified fitness professional.

6. Exercise: Bent-Over Row

Step 1: Stand with your feet shoulder-width apart and hold a dumbbell in each hand, palms facing your body. Bend your knees slightly and hinge forward at the hips, keeping your back straight and your core engaged. Let your arms hang down in front of you with a slight bend in your elbows. This is your starting position.

Step 2: Keeping your back straight and your shoulders down, pull the dumbbells towards your torso by squeezing your shoulder blades together. Focus on using your back muscles to initiate the movement, rather than relying on your arms.

Step 3: Pause at the top of the movement, making sure to keep your back straight and your core engaged. Your elbows should be pointing upwards and close to your body.

Step 4: Slowly lower the dumbbells back to the starting position, fully extending your arms and feeling a stretch in your back muscles.

Step 5: Repeat the movement for the desired number of repetitions.

Tips:

Maintain a neutral spine throughout the exercise, avoiding any rounding or arching of the back.

Keep your shoulders down and away from your ears, focusing on using your back muscles to perform the rowing motion.

Exhale as you pull the dumbbells towards your torso and inhale as you lower them back down.

Start with lighter weights to establish proper form and gradually increase the weight as you become stronger.

Use a controlled and smooth movement, avoiding any jerking or swinging of the weights.

Variations:

Barbell Bent-Over Row: Instead of using dumbbells, you can perform the bent-over row with a barbell. Hold the barbell with an overhand grip, hands slightly wider than shoulder-width apart.

Single-Arm Dumbbell Row: Perform the exercise one arm at a time, placing your non-working hand on a bench or other support for stability. This variation allows for greater focus on each side of the back.

Remember to use proper form, choose appropriate weights, and listen to your body. If you experience any pain or discomfort during the exercise, stop immediately and seek guidance from a qualified fitness professional.

7. Exercise: Bulgarian Split Squat

Step 1: Stand facing away from a bench or elevated surface, with your feet hip-width apart. Place the top of your left foot on the bench behind you, laces down.

Step 2: Take a step forward with your right foot, keeping your torso upright and core engaged. This will be your starting position.

Step 3: Lower your body by bending your right knee and hip, keeping your back straight and chest up. Descend until your right thigh is parallel to the ground, or as far as you can comfortably go.

Step 4: Pause briefly at the bottom, then push through your right heel to return to the starting position.

Step 5: Repeat for the desired number of repetitions, then switch sides and perform the exercise with your left leg forward.

Tips:

Maintain a slight forward lean with your torso to engage the glutes and hamstrings.

Keep your knee in line with your toes and avoid letting it collapse inward.

Engage your core throughout the exercise to stabilize your body.

Focus on maintaining balance and control throughout the movement.

Variations:

Goblet Bulgarian Split Squat: Hold a dumbbell or kettlebell in front of your chest to add resistance.

Bulgarian Split Squat with Rear Foot Elevated: Instead of using a bench, place your rear foot on an elevated surface like a step or box.

Note: Consult with a fitness professional or trainer if you have any concerns or limitations before attempting this exercise.

8. Exercise: Cable Row

Step 1: Stand facing a cable machine with a straight bar attachment at waist height. Hold the bar with an overhand grip, hands slightly wider than shoulder-width apart. Your feet should be shoulder-width apart, knees slightly bent, and your torso leaning slightly forward.

Step 2: Keeping your core engaged and your back straight, retract your shoulder blades and pull the bar towards your lower chest, squeezing your shoulder blades together. Keep your elbows close to your body and focus on using your back muscles to initiate the movement.

Step 3: Pause briefly at the peak of the contraction, then slowly extend your arms back to the starting position, maintaining control and tension in your back muscles.

Step 4: Repeat for the desired number of repetitions, maintaining proper form and control throughout the exercise.

Tips:

Keep your chest up and avoid rounding your back during the movement.

Focus on squeezing your shoulder blades together at the top of the movement for maximum engagement of your back muscles.

Control the weight throughout the entire range of motion, both on the pull and the release.

Adjust the weight and cable height as needed to suit your fitness level and comfort.

Variations:

Close-grip Cable Row: Use a close-grip handle or attach two single handles to the cable machine and bring your hands close together, targeting the middle back muscles.

Single-arm Cable Row: Perform the exercise with one arm at a time, focusing on maintaining stability and control.

Note: It's important to use proper form and start with an appropriate weight for your fitness level. Consult with a fitness professional or trainer if you have any concerns or limitations before attempting this exercise.

9. Exercise: Walking Lunge

Step 1: Stand tall with your feet hip-width apart and your hands on your hips or down by your sides. Take a step forward with your right foot, ensuring your knee is directly above your ankle.

Step 2: Lower your body down by bending both knees until your back knee is just above the ground and your front thigh is parallel to the floor. Keep your torso upright and engage your core for stability.

Step 3: Push through your front heel to extend your legs and bring your back leg forward, stepping into a lunge position with your left foot. Repeat the lunge movement on the opposite side.

Step 4: Continue alternating legs, walking forward with each lunge. Maintain a controlled and steady pace as you move.

Tips:

Keep your chest lifted and your shoulders relaxed throughout the movement.

Engage your core muscles to maintain balance and stability.

Step out far enough so that your front knee stays directly above your ankle and doesn't extend past your toes.

Maintain a smooth and controlled movement, avoiding any jerky or rapid motions.

To increase the difficulty, hold dumbbells in each hand or add resistance bands around your thighs.

Variations:

Reverse Lunges: Instead of stepping forward, step backward into the lunge, leading with your trailing leg.

Walking Lunges with Twist: After completing each lunge, rotate your torso towards the side of the forward leg, engaging your oblique muscles.

Walking Lunges with Overhead Reach: As you step into the lunge, raise your arms overhead, engaging your shoulder and upper back muscles.

Note: It's important to use proper form and start with an appropriate distance and pace for your fitness level. If you have any concerns or limitations, consult with a fitness professional or trainer before attempting this exercise.

10. Exercise: Kettlebell Swing

Step 1: Begin by standing with your feet shoulder-width apart, toes pointed slightly outward. Place a kettlebell on the floor in front of you.

Step 2: Squat down and grip the kettlebell handle with both hands, keeping your arms straight and your back flat. Position your hips lower than your shoulders and engage your core.

Step 3: Drive your hips forward explosively, swinging the kettlebell up to shoulder height. Use the power generated from your hips and legs to propel the kettlebell, keeping your arms relaxed and allowing the momentum to carry it upward.

Step 4: As the kettlebell reaches its highest point, squeeze your glutes and brace your core. Be sure to keep your arms straight and let the kettlebell float momentarily at the top of the swing.

Step 5: Allow the kettlebell to descend back down between your legs, hinging at the hips while maintaining a slight bend in your knees. Keep your back flat and your core engaged.

Step 6: As the kettlebell swings back between your legs, immediately drive your hips forward again to initiate the next repetition. Maintain a fluid motion, smoothly transitioning from the downswing to the upswing.

Tips:

Focus on using the power from your hips and legs to drive the kettlebell, rather than relying on your arms.

Keep your core engaged throughout the movement to maintain stability and protect your lower back.

Maintain a neutral spine position, avoiding rounding or arching your back.

Control the kettlebell with your grip, but avoid using excessive force or tension in your arms and shoulders.

Start with a lighter kettlebell and gradually increase the weight as you become more comfortable with the movement.

Variations:

Single-Arm Kettlebell Swing: Perform the same movement with one hand, gripping the kettlebell handle with a single hand.

Two-Handed Kettlebell Swing: Instead of using both hands on the handle, hold the kettlebell with both hands by the horns (sides of the handle).

Russian Kettlebell Swing: This variation involves swinging the kettlebell to shoulder height rather than overhead, focusing on the hip thrust and posterior chain engagement.

Note: It's important to use proper form and start with an appropriate weight for your fitness level. If you have any concerns or limitations, consult with a fitness professional or trainer before attempting this exercise.

11. Exercise: Jump Squat

Step 1: Start by standing with your feet shoulder-width apart, toes pointing slightly outward. Position your arms by your sides or place your hands on your hips for stability.

Step 2: Lower your body into a squat position by bending your knees and pushing your hips back. Keep your back straight, chest lifted, and your weight in your heels.

Step 3: From the squat position, explode upwards using your legs, glutes, and core muscles. Jump off the ground as high as you can, extending your arms overhead for added momentum.

Step 4: As you reach the peak of your jump, tuck your knees towards your chest and bring your arms down, crossing them in front of your body.

Step 5: Land softly on the balls of your feet, lowering your body back into the squat position to absorb the impact. Ensure your knees are aligned with your toes and your weight is in your heels.

Step 6: Repeat the exercise for the desired number of repetitions, maintaining a fluid motion and explosive power with each jump.

Tips:

Focus on maintaining proper form throughout the exercise, including a straight back, engaged core, and controlled landings.

Keep your knees aligned with your toes throughout the movement to prevent any excessive stress on your joints.

Aim to land softly and quietly, focusing on a controlled descent to minimize the impact on your joints.

Engage your glutes and leg muscles to generate power for the jump, utilizing your lower body strength.

Start with a lower intensity by performing regular squats before progressing to the jump squat.

Variations:

Single-Leg Jump Squat: Perform the same movement, but with one leg lifted off the ground. This variation adds an extra challenge to your balance and stability.

Medicine Ball Jump Squat: Hold a medicine ball against your chest as you perform the jump squat.

This adds resistance and engages your upper body muscles.

Plyometric Box Jump: Instead of jumping vertically, jump onto a plyometric box or step, ensuring a safe and stable landing surface.

Note: The jump squat is an advanced exercise that places higher demands on your lower body and joints. It's essential to have proper strength and conditioning before attempting this exercise. If you have any concerns or limitations, consult with a fitness professional or trainer before incorporating jump squats into your workout routine.

12. Exercise: Plank

Step 1: Start by positioning yourself face down on the floor, resting on your forearms and toes. Your elbows should be directly beneath your shoulders, and your forearms should be parallel to each other.

Step 2: Engage your core muscles by drawing your navel towards your spine. Your body should form a straight line from your head to your heels. Avoid sagging your hips or raising your buttocks too high.

Step 3: Hold the plank position for the desired duration, maintaining proper form and engaging your abdominal and back muscles to support your body.

Step 4: Focus on your breathing throughout the exercise. Breathe deeply and evenly, inhaling through your nose and exhaling through your mouth.

Step 5: To release the plank, gently lower your knees to the floor and rest in a kneeling position. Take a moment to stretch your arms and legs before repeating the exercise or transitioning to another movement.

Tips:

Keep your gaze down towards the floor to maintain proper alignment and avoid straining your neck.

Squeeze your glutes and thigh muscles to further engage your lower body and stabilize your hips.

Avoid holding your breath; remember to breathe naturally and continuously throughout the exercise.

Start with shorter hold times, such as 10-20 seconds, and gradually increase the duration as your core strength improves.

If the full plank position is too challenging, you can modify by performing the exercise on your knees instead of your toes.

Variations:

Side Plank: Shift your weight onto one forearm and rotate your body to the side, stacking your feet on top of each other. Extend your free arm upwards or place it on your hip. This variation targets the oblique muscles on the side of your torso.

Plank with Shoulder Taps: While in the plank position, lift one hand off the ground and tap the opposite shoulder, alternating sides. This adds an element of instability and further engages your core and shoulder muscles.

Plank Jacks: From the plank position, jump your feet out wide and then back together, similar to a jumping jack motion. This dynamic movement increases the cardiovascular challenge while maintaining core stability.

Note: The plank is a versatile exercise that targets your core muscles, including your abdominals, back muscles, and stabilizers. It can be incorporated into a variety of workout routines or used as a standalone exercise for core strength and stability. If you have any existing injuries or medical conditions, consult with a healthcare professional or fitness expert before attempting planks or any other exercise.

13. Exercise: Glute Bridge

Step 1: Start by lying on your back with your knees bent and feet flat on the floor. Place your arms by your sides with your palms facing down.

Step 2: Engage your core muscles by drawing your navel towards your spine. Press your heels into the floor and lift your hips off the ground, squeezing your glutes as you raise your body.

Step 3: Your body should form a straight line from your knees to your shoulders, with your thighs and torso parallel to the ground. Avoid arching your lower back or tilting your pelvis.

Step 4: Hold the glute bridge position for a few seconds, focusing on contracting your glute muscles and maintaining stability.

Step 5: Slowly lower your hips back down to the starting position, controlling the movement and keeping your glutes engaged throughout.

Tips:

Keep your neck relaxed and maintain a neutral spine throughout the exercise. Avoid straining your neck or shoulders by keeping them relaxed.

Exhale as you lift your hips and inhale as you lower them back down. Coordinate your breathing with the movement to enhance control and stability.

Focus on squeezing your glutes at the top of the movement to maximize muscle activation and build strength in the gluteal muscles.

If you feel any discomfort or strain in your lower back, try placing a small towel or cushion under your lower back for added support.

For an extra challenge, you can perform the exercise with your feet elevated on a stable surface such as a step or bench.

Variations:

Single-Leg Glute Bridge: Perform the glute bridge with one leg extended straight out, lifting and lowering the hips using only the supporting leg. This variation increases the activation of the glute muscles on one side at a time, providing a greater challenge to your stability and strength.

Weighted Glute Bridge: Place a weight, such as a dumbbell or barbell, on your hips as you perform the glute bridge. This adds resistance and increases the intensity of the exercise, helping to build even more strength and muscle in the glutes.

Glute Bridge March: Lift one foot off the ground and bring your knee towards your chest while maintaining the bridge position. Alternate legs in a marching motion, engaging the core and glute muscles to stabilize the hips.

Note: The glute bridge is an effective exercise for targeting and strengthening the gluteal muscles, including the gluteus maximus, medius, and minimus. It can help improve hip stability, enhance lower body strength, and alleviate lower back pain. As with any exercise, listen to your body, start with proper form and lighter resistance, and progress gradually. If you have any existing injuries or medical conditions, consult with a healthcare professional or fitness expert before attempting glute bridges or any other exercise.

14. Exercise: Seated Cable Row

Step 1: Sit on the cable row machine with your feet firmly planted on the footrests and your knees slightly bent. Grab the handles with an overhand grip, keeping your hands shoulder-width apart.

Step 2: Straighten your back, engage your core muscles, and maintain a neutral spine. Begin the exercise by pulling the handles toward your body, keeping your elbows close to your sides.

Step 3: Squeeze your shoulder blades together as you pull the handles toward your lower chest. Focus on using your back muscles to initiate the movement.

Step 4: Pause briefly at the fully contracted position, feeling the tension in your back muscles. Then, slowly release the handles and extend your arms back to the starting position, maintaining control throughout the movement.

Step 5: Repeat for the desired number of repetitions, focusing on maintaining proper form and engaging your back muscles throughout the exercise.

Note: Adjust the weight on the cable machine according to your fitness level and gradually increase the resistance as you become stronger.

15. Exercise: Standing Dumbbell Shoulder Press

Step 1: Stand with your feet shoulder-width apart, holding a dumbbell in each hand at shoulder height. Keep your core engaged and maintain a slight bend in your knees.

Step 2: Press the dumbbells upward, extending your arms fully overhead. Keep your wrists straight and your palms facing forward throughout the movement.

Step 3: As you press the dumbbells upward, exhale and engage your shoulder muscles. Avoid shrugging your shoulders or leaning back excessively.

Step 4: Pause briefly at the top of the movement, feeling the contraction in your shoulders. Maintain stability and control throughout.

Step 5: Slowly lower the dumbbells back to the starting position, bringing them back to shoulder height with control. Inhale as you lower the weights.

Step 6: Repeat for the desired number of repetitions, focusing on maintaining proper form and controlled movements.

Note: Choose a weight that challenges you but allows you to maintain proper form. If you're a beginner, start with lighter weights and gradually increase as you build strength.

3. ONE WEEK MEAL PLAN:

Day 1

Breakfast:

Spinach and mushroom omelette with whole-grain toast

Greek yogurt with mixed berries and a sprinkle of nuts

Protein pancakes topped with sliced bananas and a drizzle of honey

Snack:

Protein smoothie made with almond milk, banana, spinach, and protein powder

Hard-boiled eggs with carrot sticks

Greek yogurt with a handful of almonds

Lunch:

Grilled chicken breast with quinoa and steamed vegetables

Mixed green salad with grilled salmon and avocado

Turkey wrap with whole-wheat tortilla, lean turkey slices, lettuce, tomato, and mustard

Snack:

Cottage cheese with sliced peaches and a sprinkle of cinnamon

Rice cakes with almond butter and sliced apples

Veggie sticks with hummus

Dinner:

Baked salmon with roasted sweet potatoes and steamed broccoli

Lean beef stir-fry with brown rice and mixed vegetables

Grilled chicken with quinoa salad and grilled asparagus

Snack:

Protein bar or protein shake

Greek yogurt with mixed berries and a sprinkle of granola

Raw nuts and seeds mix

Day 2

Breakfast:

Protein-packed smoothie bowl with unsweetened almond milk, frozen berries, spinach, and a scoop of protein powder, topped with sliced almonds and chia seeds

Scrambled eggs with sautéed vegetables (such as bell peppers, onions, and zucchini) and a side of whole-grain toast

Quinoa breakfast bowl with cooked quinoa, Greek yogurt, mixed fruits, and a drizzle of honey

Snack:

Protein-rich energy balls made with rolled oats, almond butter, protein powder, and dark chocolate chips

Celery sticks with almond butter and raisins

Cottage cheese with sliced cucumbers and cherry tomatoes

Lunch:

Grilled chicken or tofu salad with mixed greens, cherry tomatoes, cucumbers, avocado, and a light vinaigrette dressing

Turkey or veggie burger on a whole-grain bun, topped with lettuce, tomato, and pickles, served with sweet potato fries

Quinoa-stuffed bell peppers with lean ground turkey, black beans, corn, and spices

Snack:

Greek yogurt parfait with layers of Greek yogurt, fresh berries, and a sprinkle of granola

Sliced apple with almond butter

Edamame beans lightly seasoned with sea salt

Dinner:

Grilled salmon with roasted asparagus and quinoa pilaf

Lean beef or tofu stir-fry with a variety of colorful vegetables, served over brown rice

Baked chicken breast with steamed broccoli and a side of sweet potato mash

Snack:

Protein-rich chocolate smoothie made with almond milk, cocoa powder, a scoop of protein powder, and a handful of spinach

Raw mixed nuts and dried fruit trail mix

Vegetable sticks with tzatziki dip

Day 3

Breakfast:

Omelette with egg whites, spinach, mushrooms, and feta cheese, served with a side of whole-grain toast

Overnight oats made with rolled oats, almond milk, Greek yogurt, chia seeds, and topped with fresh berries and a drizzle of honey

Whole-grain pancakes topped with sliced bananas, a dollop of Greek yogurt, and a sprinkle of crushed walnuts

Snack:

Veggie sticks (carrots, celery, bell peppers) with hummus

Protein smoothie made with almond milk, frozen mixed berries, spinach, and a scoop of protein powder

Rice cakes topped with almond butter and sliced strawberries

Lunch:

Grilled chicken or tempeh salad with mixed greens, cherry tomatoes, cucumbers, avocado, and a lemon-tahini dressing

Quinoa bowl with roasted vegetables (such as sweet potatoes, Brussels sprouts, and bell peppers) and a drizzle of balsamic glaze

Lentil soup with a side of mixed green salad and a whole-grain roll

Snack:

Greek yogurt with a sprinkle of granola and fresh blueberries

Hard-boiled eggs with a side of cherry tomatoes

Whole-grain crackers with almond butter and sliced apples

Dinner:

Grilled shrimp skewers with a quinoa and vegetable medley

Baked salmon with steamed broccoli and a quinoa pilaf

Turkey or tofu lettuce wraps with a side of brown rice

Snack:

Protein bars made with oats, protein powder, nut butter, and dried fruit

Cottage cheese with sliced peaches and a drizzle of honey

Roasted chickpeas with sea salt and paprika

Day 4

Breakfast:

Greek yogurt parfait layered with mixed berries, granola, and a drizzle of honey

Scrambled eggs with sautéed vegetables (such as bell peppers, onions, and spinach) served with whole-grain toast

Protein-packed smoothie bowl topped with sliced bananas, almond butter, and a sprinkle of chia seeds

Snack:

Apple slices with almond butter

Roasted edamame with a sprinkle of sea salt

Cottage cheese with sliced cucumbers and a dash of black pepper

Lunch:

Grilled chicken or tofu stir-fry with a variety of colorful vegetables (such as broccoli, snap peas, carrots, and bell peppers) and served over brown rice or quinoa

Quinoa and black bean salad with diced tomatoes, corn, avocado, and a lime-cilantro dressing

Whole-grain wrap filled with lean turkey, hummus, spinach, and sliced tomatoes

Snack:

Homemade protein balls made with oats, almond butter, protein powder, and dark chocolate chips

A handful of mixed nuts and dried fruit

Celery sticks with peanut butter and raisins (also known as "ants on a log")

Dinner:

Grilled lean steak or portobello mushrooms with roasted sweet potatoes and steamed asparagus

Baked chicken breast with quinoa and roasted Brussels sprouts

Spaghetti squash with turkey meatballs and marinara sauce, served with a side salad

Snack:

Greek yogurt with a sprinkle of cinnamon and sliced almonds

Rice cakes with avocado and smoked salmon

Roasted kale chips seasoned with olive oil and sea salt

Day 5

Breakfast:

Veggie omelette made with egg whites, spinach, mushrooms, and low-fat cheese

Protein pancake stack topped with fresh berries and a dollop of Greek yogurt

Overnight oats prepared with almond milk, chia seeds, and sliced almonds, topped with diced mango and a drizzle of honey

Snack:

Roasted chickpeas seasoned with paprika and cumin

Turkey or chicken lettuce wraps with a squeeze of fresh lemon juice

Protein smoothie made with almond milk, frozen berries, spinach, and a scoop of protein powder

Lunch:

Grilled salmon with quinoa and roasted vegetables (such as zucchini, bell peppers, and carrots)

Quinoa-stuffed bell peppers with ground turkey, black beans, corn, and salsa

Whole-grain pasta tossed with grilled chicken, cherry tomatoes, and pesto sauce

Snack:

Sliced cucumber with hummus for dipping

Cottage cheese with sliced peaches and a sprinkle of cinnamon

Homemade trail mix with almonds, walnuts, dried cranberries, and dark chocolate chunks

Dinner:

Baked cod with roasted sweet potatoes and a side of steamed broccoli

Grilled chicken breast with a side of quinoa and sautéed kale

Lentil curry with brown rice and a mixed green salad

Snack:

Rice cakes topped with mashed avocado and sliced tomatoes

Protein-rich Greek yogurt with a handful of mixed berries

Roasted seaweed sheets for a light and crunchy snack

Day 6

Breakfast:

Greek yogurt parfait layered with mixed berries, granola, and a drizzle of honey

Whole-grain toast topped with mashed avocado, sliced hard-boiled eggs, and a sprinkle of black pepper

Protein-packed smoothie bowl made with frozen banana, spinach, almond milk, and a scoop of protein powder, topped with sliced almonds and shredded coconut

Snack:

Apple slices with almond butter

Homemade protein bars made with oats, nut butter, and protein powder

Veggie sticks (carrots, celery, bell peppers) with a side of Greek yogurt dip

Lunch:

Grilled chicken or tofu stir-fry with a variety of colorful vegetables (broccoli, bell peppers, snap peas) and served over brown rice or quinoa

Quinoa salad with mixed greens, cherry tomatoes, cucumber, feta cheese, and a lemon-herb dressing

Turkey or veggie burger with whole-grain bun, lettuce, tomato, and avocado, served with sweet potato fries

Snack:

High-protein cottage cheese with sliced pineapple and a sprinkle of cinnamon

Rice cakes topped with almond butter and banana slices

Roasted edamame for a crunchy and protein-rich snack

Dinner:

Grilled steak with roasted Brussels sprouts and a quinoa pilaf

Baked chicken breast with steamed asparagus and roasted potatoes

Shrimp or tofu stir-fry with a mix of colorful vegetables (snow peas, carrots, bok choy) and served over whole-grain noodles or brown rice

Snack:

Greek yogurt with a sprinkle of granola and a handful of mixed nuts

Sliced pear with a spread of almond butter and a drizzle of honey

Homemade protein balls made with oats, peanut butter, and chocolate chips

Day 7

Breakfast:

Veggie omelet made with egg whites, spinach, mushrooms, and feta cheese

Whole-grain pancakes topped with sliced bananas and a drizzle of maple syrup

Quinoa breakfast bowl with mixed berries, almond milk, and a sprinkle of chia seeds

Snack:

Greek yogurt with a handful of mixed nuts and a sprinkle of cinnamon

Rice cakes with avocado spread and smoked salmon

Roasted chickpeas for a crunchy and protein-rich snack

Lunch:

Grilled salmon or tofu with a side of roasted vegetables (such as zucchini, bell peppers, and onions) and quinoa

Spinach salad with grilled chicken, strawberries, almonds, and a balsamic vinaigrette dressing

Turkey or veggie wrap with whole-grain tortilla, lettuce, tomato, cucumber, and a smear of hummus

Snack:

Celery sticks with almond butter and raisins

Hard-boiled eggs with a sprinkle of sea salt

Homemade protein muffins made with oats, bananas, and your choice of protein powder

Dinner:

Baked cod with steamed broccoli and quinoa

Grilled chicken or tempeh with roasted sweet potatoes and sautéed kale

Beef or vegetable stir-fry with a mix of colorful vegetables (such as bell peppers, snap peas, and carrots) and served over brown rice

Snack:

Cottage cheese with sliced peaches and a drizzle of honey

Rice cakes topped with hummus and cucumber slices

Mixed berries with a dollop of Greek yogurt and a sprinkle of granola

These meal ideas provide a balance of nutrients, including lean proteins, complex carbohydrates, and healthy fats, to support muscle development, provide sustained energy, and promote overall well-being.

Remember to adjust portion sizes based on your individual needs and goals, and consider incorporating a variety of fruits, vegetables, and whole grains into your meals.

It's important to note that these meal ideas are general suggestions, and it's always recommended to consult with a registered dietitian or nutritionist for personalized advice. They can help create a tailored meal plan that suits your specific dietary requirements, preferences, and fitness goals.

Please remember that while a balanced diet is essential for overall health and fitness, individual nutritional needs may vary. It's crucial to listen to your body, fuel it appropriately, and make adjustments as needed to support your unique journey.

4. A PROGRESSIVE TRACKER:

A progress tracker is a valuable tool to monitor and measure your achievements throughout your fitness journey. It helps you stay accountable, track your progress, and make necessary adjustments to your training and nutrition plan. Here are some key components of a progress tracker:

Measurement and Weigh-In: Record your body measurements (such as waist, hips, chest, and thighs) and weigh yourself regularly. This provides a baseline to track changes in body composition over time.

Fitness Assessments: Conduct regular fitness assessments to measure your strength, endurance, flexibility, and other relevant fitness parameters. This can include exercises like push-ups, sit-ups, squats, and timed runs.

Photos: Take progress photos at regular intervals, such as every four to six weeks. These photos can help visually track changes in your physique, muscle definition, and overall body composition.

Workout Logs: Keep a detailed log of your workouts, including exercises performed, sets, reps, and weights lifted. This allows you to track your strength progress and identify areas where you can push yourself further.

Nutrition Diary: Maintain a food diary or use a mobile app to track your daily food intake. Record your meals, snacks, and portion sizes to gain insights into your nutrition habits and make adjustments if necessary.

Energy Levels and Mood: Note how you feel before, during, and after workouts, as well as throughout the day. This helps you understand how different factors, such as sleep, stress, and nutrition, affect your energy levels and overall well-being.

Goal Setting and Reflection: Set specific, measurable goals and regularly review and adjust them based on your progress. Reflect on your achievements and challenges to stay motivated and identify areas for improvement.

Personal Records (PRs): Keep a record of your personal bests or PRs for different exercises, such as your maximum weight lifted in a particular lift or the fastest time completed in a cardio workout. This allows you to track improvements and set new goals.

Weekly or Monthly Summaries: Summarize your progress at regular intervals, such as weekly or monthly. This can include a brief overview of your achievements, challenges faced, and any adjustments made to your training or nutrition plan.

Notes and Observations: Use the progress tracker as a journal to jot down any observations, breakthroughs, or obstacles you encounter along the way. This provides valuable insights and helps you learn from your experiences.

Remember, consistency is key when using a progress tracker. Regularly update your measurements, record your workouts, and review your progress to make informed decisions and stay motivated on your fitness journey.